How to Write Health Sciences Papers, Dissertations and Theses

Shane A. Thomas BA(Hons) DipPublicPolicy PhD

Adjunct Professor, Australian Institute of Primary Care, La Trobe University, Melbourne, Australia

Adjunct Professor, School of Nursing, Deakin University, Melbourne, Australia

Visiting Principal Research Fellow, School of Social Work, University of Melbourne, Melbourne, Australia

Senior Fellow, School of Behavioural Science, University of Melbourne, Melbourne, Australia

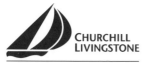
CHURCHILL LIVINGSTONE

EDINBURGH LONDON NEW YORK PHILADELPHIA ST LOUIS SYDNEY TORONTO 2000

CHURCHILL LIVINGSTONE
An imprint of Harcourt Publishers Limited

© Harcourt Publishers Limited 2000

 is a registered trademark of Harcourt Publishers Limited

The right of Shane Thomas to be identified as author of this work has been asserted by him in accordance with the Copyright, Designs and Patents Act 1988

First published 2000

0 443 06283 8

British Library Cataloguing in Publication Data
A catalogue record for this book is available from the British Library

Library of Congress Cataloging in Publication Data
A catalog record for this book is available from the Library of Congress

The
publisher's
policy is to use
**paper manufactured
from sustainable forests**

Printed in China

How to Write Health Sciences Papers, Dissertations and Theses

WITHDRAWN

*For my darling son Liam Patrick Browning Thomas
and his mother and my mother*

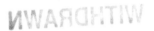

For Churchill Livingstone

Editorial Director, Health Professions: Mary Law
Project Development Manager: Dinah Thom
Project Manager: Jane Shanks
Design Direction: George Ajayi

Contents

Foreword

I am pleased to be given the opportunity to write the foreword for *How to Write Health Sciences Papers, Dissertations and Theses*. Professor Thomas's book is not just another academic piece on how to write health sciences theses and papers. It complements currently available codes and guidelines on the subject, but it also challenges some of the current practices in research training for health scientists. For instance, in the very first stage of planning a research project, questions are raised on the sensibility of appointing academic staff based on seniority for supervision. From the student's perspective, choosing the 'right' supervisor is one of the first major decisions; it is indeed a crucial factor for a successful outcome. Professor Thomas provides examples on how to go about selecting the right supervisor.

The management of supervisor–student conflict is another issue which often goes unmentioned in the existing codes and guidelines. This book provides examples on how to deal with the conflict whilst continuing to carry on one's work. It sets down strategies which until now have remained largely unwritten, or which are often considered as 'commonsense' and so in consequence can sometimes be overlooked because often simple approaches are not always valued.

Naturally both students and supervisors would like to achieve successful outcomes in the preparation of the final thesis, but it is unlikely that such outcomes will be secured without the commitment and determination of both parties. Professor Thomas shows that the production of a thesis is not simply a writing process; rather, it is the end result of an onerous sequence of tasks performed in various settings. In describing these tasks he places emphasis on the crucial structural components of health sciences theses and papers. The partnership between the student and the supervisor(s) is examined, and the need for developing a thesis management plan from the start is advocated.

This interesting book is written in a user-friendly style and is suitable for use by both students and supervisors. It will provide an invaluable guide for the research student in the health sciences and should be read before embarking upon any major research project. Unfinished work by students and supervisors in higher education is a major issue. This book will make a positive contribution towards the successful completion of research work and reporting.

Melbourne 2000   Professor Lerma CM Ung

Preface

One of the remarkable features of health sciences education in western countries since the 1980s has been the influx of this education into the universities from the craft guild-like structures previously entrusted with professional training. I have had the privilege of observing these changes first-hand during the almost 2 decades in which I have been involved in health sciences education. In 1988, the health sciences institute at which I had been a staff member for 11 years amalgamated with a large university, thus providing direct access for the enrolment of students in Doctoral programmes for the first time.

During my academic career, I have supervised 24 Doctoral and Masters degrees by research students and about 100 Honours and Diploma students to the successful completion of their degrees in the health sciences. I have learnt a great deal from my students and I hope that the reverse may also be true.

I must also say that as someone who has been involved in the academic administration of higher degree examinations for some time, and also as a regular examiner myself, I have seen many examples where students have made basic and avoidable mistakes in the presentation of their theses and the conduct of their research programmes. I see an unfinished or unnecessarily delayed degree as a huge waste of time for the student and the academic staff involved and as a large opportunity for the advancement of knowledge lost. Frankly, I am unimpressed with the design and performance of some of the current systems of research training for health scientists, although much promise remains. The attrition rates for research students in terms of unfinished degrees in the UK, USA and Australia are far too high.

Although my colleagues from other disciplines may disagree, I think that in the area of the health and medical sciences, such attrition is an especially important loss to the community. Much of what we do in the health and medical sciences has the potential to assist the human condition and to avoid and minimise suffering in ways not as readily available to other disciplines.

Thus, this book is an attempt to assist students and their supervisors working in the health sciences to complete their research studies at the Honours and higher degree levels. My hope is that it is of use to others involved in health sciences research.

I would like to thank my colleague and friend Steve Polgar, with whom I have had a very successful working partnership for 15 years. Steve and I first co-wrote our *Introduction to Research in the Health Sciences* text almost 10 years ago. Yet the excitement still remains. I also wish to thank Colette Browning for her academic and personal encouragement in producing this material and for co-authoring on our son Liam.

I thank Steve and Colette for their comments on my tortured English and fractured concepts. I also thank all of my students. It has been fun.

Melbourne, 2000   Shane Thomas

Overview of this book

INTRODUCTION

In the western world, health scientists have seen a remarkable transition in their disciplines since the 1980s. Many have made the transition from craft guild models of training and accreditation structures conducted in separate institutes or hospitals to mainstream universities and colleges. The usual entry to health sciences practice for new entrants now involves the completion of an undergraduate degree. Increasing numbers of health scientists are now also studying for Honours, Masters and Doctoral degrees. An integral component of these degrees is the research thesis.

The production of the thesis requires the design and execution of a robust research programme and then its reporting in the form of the thesis. The two tasks of performing and then reporting the research are, of course, strongly linked. They therefore need to be discussed in a way that recognises this link. Texts such as Polgar & Thomas (1995) *Introduction to Research in the Health Sciences* have been widely adopted in undergraduate health sciences training in the UK, Canada and Australia. Such texts emphasise the design aspects of health sciences research but, while they contain some discussion of scientific reporting, they are of insufficient scope to address the practical requirements of the health scientist who is confronted with the task of producing a research thesis.

The purpose of this book is to help health sciences research students and their supervisors to complete the task of the production of the research thesis. It includes many templates and ideas designed to assist the student and the supervisor with their respective tasks.

AN OVERVIEW OF THE HEALTH SCIENCES THESIS STRUCTURE

The health sciences thesis typically follows a well-prescribed overall structure. It contains the following elements:

1. Thesis title page
2. Table of Contents
3. Declaration of authorship
4. List of publications arising from thesis
5. List of Figures and Tables
6. Acknowledgements
7. Dedication
8. Abstract
9. Introduction and literature review
8. Methodology (one for each study or sub-study)
10. Results and discussion chapters (one for each study or sub-study)
11. Conclusions
12. References
13. Appendices.

The substance of the thesis appears in the abstract, introduction and literature review, methodology, results and discussion chapters and conclusions chapters. However, the production of a research thesis is not simply a writing task. It is the culmination of an often arduous and lengthy sequence of tasks performed in academic, clinical and community contexts. Many people are involved in these tasks. This book reflects both a focus on the writing tasks and the research context in which theses are written.

Chapter 2 of this text is concerned with issues arising from the supervision of the student in the research programme and the thesis. It is noted that the research on attrition rates for research students in the UK, USA and Australia shows that many students do not complete their ultimate goal of submitting a thesis for examination. The factors associated with student success and failure are reviewed. It is argued that supervisor quality and the approach taken by the supervisor can have a major impact upon the student's success. The issues of meetings between student and supervisor and how to maximise their utility are discussed. Also the necessity for supervisors to ensure that students have access to the resources required to complete their research is emphasised. Strategies for dealing with student–supervisor and supervisor–supervisor conflict are proposed.

Chapter 3 presents a number of strategies for the facilitation of the writing of the thesis. The development of a writing plan is shown as well as how to get started and how to overcome problems such as writer's block.

In Chapter 4, the crucial issue of determining the appropriate scope and size of the research programme and the thesis is discussed. Information concerning typical thesis size parameters is presented together with suggestions as to the typical extent of the research programme, including the number and the size of studies reported within it.

The introduction and literature review of the thesis is discussed in Chapter 5. A three-stage writing process is presented for the production of the literature review consisting of description, critique and integration. This process is illustrated through the construction of components of the review in order that students may readily adopt this process with their own material.

Chapter 6 presents methods for literature searching and management including computer-based techniques.

Chapter 7 describes how to write the thesis methodology. An important feature of this chapter is the construction of the methodological defence for the thesis. Examples of such defences are provided to assist readers in the construction of their own.

The procedures and principles involved in obtaining ethical clearance for research projects is discussed in Chapter 8. The concept of informed consent is also reviewed.

Chapter 9 discusses how to write the results and discussion of the thesis. This is a core component of this book. It covers issues such as the design of results tables and figures, issues in the reporting of statistical analyses and how to integrate the results and discussion. Both qualitative and quantitative examples are given. Extensive use of examples is designed to assist in the application of these principles to the reader's own thesis.

In Chapter 10, the thesis conclusion is discussed. A procedure termed 'deconstruction' is described. This procedure greatly facilitates the rapid production of a draft of the conclusion. It is argued that the conclusion should consist of several components: a summary of the outcomes of the literature review culminating in the research questions, an overview of the research programme and methodology used to address the research questions, the major findings of the thesis and how they integrate with previous work and future work.

Chapter 11 describes in detail how to construct the abstract of the thesis, while Chapter 12 deals with the final production of the thesis including all the components such as title pages, acknowledgements, appendices, etc. This information is liberally supported by detailed examples. The purpose of this chapter is to give the student unambiguous advice about how to take the final draft to the submission stage.

The examination process for the thesis is described in Chapter 13. The thesis submission process, how the examination is normally conducted and how to deal with examiners' reports are all discussed.

Issues arising from the publication of work from the thesis are discussed in Chapter 14. The conventions that govern academic authorship are discussed, along with the advantages of publication before the completion of the thesis. Various methods of publication are discussed together with their respective merits.

Chapter 15 is a very short chapter designed to assist with the last sentence of the thesis. A thesis preparation checklist is provided as an Appendix at the end of the book as an aid to the process of thesis preparation.

The book can be read in a linear sequence. Indeed, the order of presentation corresponds to the usual order of activities involved in the construction of a thesis. For example, the abstract to the thesis is the last substantive section of the thesis that is written and this is reflected in the placement of this chapter in the text. However, for the student or supervisor who is having problems with a particular aspect of the thesis, this text has been written in such a way as to permit direct entry to that section in a stand-alone manner.

2

Supervision and the chances of success

This chapter is concerned with the key relationship between the supervisor(s) and the research student. It commences with a discussion of student completion rates in research degrees and how the supervision process may facilitate or hinder the completion of the degree.

STUDENT COMPLETION RATES (WHAT ARE THE ODDS?)

One of the least discussed aspects of student research is the progression and completion rates for students involved in research degree programmes and coursework programmes that involve a research thesis. These rates have been found to vary with the level of the degree. While most Honours or Diploma students complete their year of study and complete the research thesis, higher degree students, perhaps because of the length and difficulty of their programmes, are less likely to complete at all and often take extended periods to do so.

The issue of completion rates in research degrees is of paramount importance to research students and supervisors, but there are significant gaps in the available research. The conduct of research into completion rates engenders a number of procedural and methodological challenges.

Because postgraduate research degrees take so long to complete, the research also takes a long time to do. For example, if one wanted to do a prospective study of the progress of research students, perhaps 5 years of student cohorts would provide a satisfactory basis for this type of study. Since completion for part-time candidates may take 10 years for a PhD, then one would have to wait 15 years for the final results. Of course, doing the research retrospectively shortens the data collection time interval but, as we all know, retrospective designs can have some major difficulties.

The lengthy time intervals for the completion of research degrees also create interpretational difficulties for this type of study. Even the most current research student completion rate data is, in a sense, a history lesson, because the students who have just completed may have started 10 years ago. No-one can know with certainty what the completion rates for candidates starting today will be. Academia in most English-speaking countries is in a period of major change, rendering 10-year-old research about circumstances prevailing then to be dated indeed.

Bearing in mind these precautionary considerations, let us turn to the few major studies that are available on this topic in the USA, UK and Australia. As will be seen below, while the systems for research training differ from country to country, there is a high communality in the findings of this research.

In the USA, there are currently several large-scale research programmes under way concerning research doctorate programmes. The Association of American Universities Association of Graduate Schools is conducting a major research programme aimed at studying, among other matters, patterns of retention, completion and time to degree across various PhD fields. Unfortunately, the project has not been in operation for a sufficient period to provide useful data as yet.

Also in the USA, the Office of Scientific and Engineering Personnel of the National Academy of Sciences has sponsored several major studies of attrition and completion rates of research doctorates. The report *The Path to the Ph.D.* (Office of Scientific and Engineering Personnel, 1997) notes that some institutions have reported research doctorate attrition rates between 50 and 65%, but that most are not in a position to provide accurate data concerning the actual attrition rates for their students. This report focuses on the difficulties associated with the development of common reporting standards so that rates are comparable.

Notwithstanding these interpretational issues, the attrition rates reported within this study are quite high. The same Office has also released a study of the time it takes for students to complete research doctorates, but it is now quite dated (Office of Scientific and Engineering Personnel, 1990). The study investigated the effects of family background, student attributes, financial aid, institutional variables and market forces upon completion times, over an extended time period from 1967 to 1986. A complex pattern of interrelationships between these factors and completion times and rates was found in the study. However, the most notable feature was strong growth in the length of candidature periods. The study concluded that 'it now takes longer to complete a doctoral degree than at any previous time in this century' (p. 2).

Some brave US institutions publish their data concerning research student completion rates. For example, the University of California at San Diego has released PhD completion and attrition rates for student who entered PhD programmes between 1981 and 1986, broken down by department (available at www.ogr.ucsd.edu/graddata/coh5yr.htm). The proportion of students who had completed their degrees 10 years after initial enrolment was 57%. The discipline of the students was a major predictor of these rates, with, for example, students from history, philosophy and literature having an aggregate 10-year completion rate of 39%. The corresponding figure for basic sciences was 68%. Psychology had a completion rate of 71% and anthropology's rate was 44%. For individual departments the lowest rate of completion was 20% for one department, whereas another department had a 100% completion rate for its students. Interestingly, the size of the enrolment in the departments was correlated $r = + 0.41$ with 10-year completion rates. In other words, the more research students enrolled in a department, the more likely that department was to have a higher student completion rate. While these data relate to one university only, this is a very large study, involving data for 1553 PhD students.

A British study is reported by Booth & Satchell (1996) in which they analysed the outcomes of the 1986/7 National Survey of 1980 Graduates and Diplomates. The survey sample comprised 484 people who had embarked on a PhD in 1980. At the time of the survey 66% of the respondents had completed their degrees. The researchers modelled the impacts of various factors upon completion rates and times. The factors studied included gender, student quality and area of research. PhD students in the arts and languages had significantly lower rates of completion than those in the social sciences, who in turn had lower rates than those enrolled in the basic sciences. Female PhD students were more likely to withdraw than male students, and took longer to complete their degrees. The researchers' models also showed that, as duration of candidature increased, so did the probability of withdrawal from candidature.

In Australia, there are only patchy data available concerning research student completion rates. The Federal Department of Employment Training and Youth Affairs oversees Higher Education in Australia and provides comprehensive reports concerning numbers of student completions. However, because it does not maintain unit record data, it is usually not in a position to report upon completion rates. Nevertheless, in the Government Green Paper concerning the training of researchers that was released in June 1999, some reference was made to this matter (Department of Education, Training and Youth Affairs, 1999). It is noted in the report that in 1997, the attrition rate for all higher degree research courses in Australia was 34%, although the basis for this calculation is not clearly specified. It is further noted that analysis of the 1992 enrolment cohort found that only 38% of students had completed their studies after 6 years. This figure includes both Masters students (for which in Australia the usual full-time and part-time completion times are regulated to be 2 and 4 years, respectively) and PhD students (for which in Australia the usual full-time completion time is regulated to be a maximum of 3.5 years, with a wide variation in part-time rates between institutions). If only 38% of all research students including Masters students within this group had completed after 6 years, then this implies very low 6-year completion rates for Australian PhD candidates. This is because after 6 years the degree regulations at most Australian institutions would have crystallised into either completion or failure for the Masters students.

It is interesting that, despite the different systems of student training in operation in the different English-speaking countries, there is a common finding that the attrition rates for research students are quite high, but also with major variability within disciplines and departments.

Why, then, are the rates overall so low, and why is there so much variability? In our clinical settings, if we killed 65% of our patient, there would be an outcry. Yet as we have seen, some departments manage to have 80% of their students fail to complete their research degrees. It is sobering to consider that it could well be that the successful completions from within those departments stem from a small number or perhaps just one of the academic staff. What a waste of human potential!

Thus, there is cause for concern about the completion of research degrees. Indeed, this loss was one of the reasons that motivated the production of this text. One of the prime functions of this book is to assist students in producing their theses and in avoiding the pitfalls that can impede their progress in this task.

SUPERVISION ARRANGEMENTS

In universities modelled on the British university system, including the Australian system, it is the norm to have only one or perhaps two supervisors involved in supervision of the research student. With Honours degrees, it is almost always only one supervisor who is involved. Those universities in, or modelled on, the US system typically employ a supervisory panel with a principal supervisor and a number of associate supervisors who serve on the supervision panel. Supervision is important in any system, but in a single supervisor situation as in a British or British-modelled university, the quality of the supervision is even more crucial for student progression and ultimate completion. In a panel supervision arrangement as employed in the USA it is possible to access a range of expert people. If any one supervisor is unsatisfactory then the homeostatic mechanisms with the other supervisors can come into force. In a sole supervisor situation, if the supervisor is a 'dud', then this can be a very serious problem for students ānd for their chances of successful completion of the degree.

The ensuing discussion is unlikely to win friends among my academic colleagues but I feel obliged to be honest and direct to the student reader. It is necessary to acknowledge that some academic staff have very low, sometimes zero, research student completion rates. While there are many alternative explanations for this fact other than supervisor quality, I am of the view that, in the face of a long-term trend of lack of successful completion of students, one must look to this factor. How, then, can one determine the supervisor's track record in student completion?

I have found the seniority of appointment of the academic staff member to be an unreliable guide to student completion rates. It might reasonably be expected that good student completion rates would be an attribute expected (some might say demanded) of senior academics. This is not always the case. In the academic environment it is often on the basis of personal research activity, not student research activity, that promotion is provided. Some senior academics with 25-year careers have graduated only a handful of Honours, Masters and/or Doctoral students over their entire careers. On the other hand, some have graduated a great many. Perhaps this is the academic corollary of the saying 'If you want a job done, give it to a busy person'. But not too busy to see you!

How, then, are you to discover the supervisory high performers? One way is to study the last few years of the university and departmental research reports and see the names of the students who have graduated, i.e. those who have successfully completed their degrees. Talk to them. Find out who supervised them. Most university libraries and departments maintain collections of their higher degree theses. Departmental libraries also usually house the Honours theses. Have a browse through them and see who supervised them. Unfortunately, this procedure does not tell you who did not hand in their thesis. It is also possible that the names of the academic staff who do not appear in the list of completed thesis supervisors are not there because they did not supervise any students. Lack of opportunity is not an indication of failure to succeed.

If you are considering a particular supervisor and are in personal contact with him or her, you could ask if you could borrow some copies of the theses that he or she has supervised so that you can check the standard you will need to reach and the topics they have studied.

Newcomer academic staff should not be rejected as prospective supervisors. Although there may be some costs associated with supervisory inexperience, youthful enthusiasm and vigour can also be very useful. Further, the academics with large numbers of completed students all had their first student. You may be the first born in a long dynasty of students supervised to completion by that person. It may be better to try an enthusiastic inexperienced person rather than a person with a long but unproductive supervisory track record. However, if there is an experienced person available with a good track record of student completion, then clearly that person should be given every consideration if he or she is available and you 'click' with each other.

The selection of a research thesis supervisor is a business arrangement. You would not hire a plumber with dodgy credentials whom no-one else had hired and whose work you had not seen. It pays to be well researched and well informed about the person with whom you are going to entrust a key part of your career. Go and meet with the possible prospects. As discussed later, you do not have to like them or vice versa, but they need to be able to deliver for you. Past performance is an impeccable guide to future performance.

In some cases, I have heard of situations where students are allocated to academic staff, without student input. While this can work, I think choice is a much better approach. Having chosen or having been allocated to a supervisor, what happens during this dialogue?

THE STUDENT–SUPERVISOR DIALOGUE

The relationship between the research student and the supervisor has no direct analogue in other facets of everyday life. In the case of a PhD candidature, the student and supervisor may meet 100 or more times during the candidature with the sole purpose of assisting and directing the student with the research programme and the production of the thesis. For other degrees the dialogue is more compressed. It is typical for an Honours candidate to meet their supervisor on a weekly basis and sometimes more frequently for the year of their studies, involving perhaps 40 meetings during the candidature. Enormous amounts of time are invested by both parties to the supervision and thesis production tasks if each contributes as he or she ought.

Much has been written about the necessity for a good relationship between the student and the supervisor(s). I sometimes feel that because of the imprecision of the term 'relationship' it can be confused with friendship. Certainly the basic elements for friendship need to be there for the relationship to work well: basic respect for each other, an ability to see the other person's point of view, a desire to spend time jointly on the completion of the required tasks and a love of the work. However, the relationship is a working one and it is the work efficiency and effectiveness that needs to be the focus. Academic or collegial friendship is a bonus on top of an effective working association. It is helpful but not compulsory for the smooth flow of the degree.

A number of issues need to be addressed to ensure an effective student–supervisor relationship and work programme. These include consideration of the meeting frequency between students and supervisors, the determination of meeting purpose and content, the preparation of written work for meetings, student access to resources to support their research and the management of conflict should it arise.

MEETING FREQUENCY BETWEEN STUDENTS AND SUPERVISORS

Most universities have guidelines concerning the minimum acceptable meeting frequency between students and supervisors. In the case of higher degree students these regulations generally state that monthly meetings are the minimum requirement. In the case of Honours students, if the meetings were monthly, then the candidature would be over before the parties had introduced themselves! In this instance a 2-week interval is probably the maximum that should wisely elapse between contacts. At the outset of the candidature this issue of meeting frequency and length should be discussed. Some flexibility in meeting schedules is important. For example, during the thesis data collection phase, there is probably a lessened requirement for meetings. While the thesis is being drafted, provided the student has detailed instructions, then there is also probably a lessened requirement for face-to-face meetings. During the design phase and the determination of the research questions, the meetings should be more frequent. However, lengthy intervals between meetings is not a good idea.

MEETING PURPOSE AND CONTENT

From the supervisor(s)' point of view, there are other reasons for meeting than simply to address the mechanics of the work programme. Many students worry unduly about a variety of things about their research. Am I good enough to complete the degree? Has someone else already performed this work and published it in an obscure journal somewhere that only the examiners will know about? Is the work good enough? Am I tall enough?

Part of the function of the student supervisor meeting is for the supervisor to maintain the student in the optimal part of the Yerkes–Dodson performance–anxiety curve. That is, one should not remove anxiety completely, because a bit of fear of failure is always good for one's performance. It has kept me going for a couple of decades. However, it needs to be kept under control. Sensitivity for student problems outside the research programme is, of course, part of being a human being and a professional, but if professional help is required for personal problems, then it is best for the student to seek it from a third party rather than from the supervisor. Your boss should not be your therapist.

Both parties need to come to the meeting in a reasonable state of organisation. At the outset of the meeting, a brief discussion should be held to determine the goals of the meeting, i.e. the agenda. The student should provide a short report on activities undertaken since the last meeting and both student and supervisor should report on the outcomes of the tasks they agreed to complete at the last meeting. At the conclusion of the meeting, it is important than both parties record and understand what it is that is to occur before the next meeting.

To facilitate this process, I maintain separate folders for each of my students in which I file their drafts, any correspondence between us and notes concerning what we have agreed to do. It is similar to a medical record. I have found this to be an invaluable resource in order to resolve any issues that may arise concerning the candidature. I suggest that students maintain similar records.

PREPARING WRITTEN WORK FOR THE SUPERVISOR

When all is said and done, the research thesis is a written document of some considerable length. It is wise to spread the production of this document over the candidature rather than to prepare it all at the end. In addition to draft sections of the thesis, other documentation may be required. For example, most research requires ethics clearance from the relevant bodies (see the discussion in Chapter 8 for more details). Thus the student should be preparing written work on a regular basis for academic input from the supervisor. From the supervisor's viewpoint, in most instances I have found it helpful to write the students a formal letter giving my advice concerning the material they have presented, as well as presenting the advice verbally in the meeting. I think this formality is helpful as tricks of memory can be a problem with detailed technical material. It also prevents me from committing one of the cardinal supervisory sins – providing contradictory advice with oneself! Advising students to journey in one direction and then 6 months later to proceed in the other direction drives them crazy, with good reason. They may begin to doubt the quality of the navigation.

One of the areas of contention that can develop between students and supervisors is the return of comments on drafted materials. Naturally students are keen to proceed with their studies. Sometimes this keenness can develop into unrealistic expectations on the part of the student. I have had students take a year to draft some materials and then, without a hint of embarrassment, explain how convenient it would be if I could have my comments back early next week because they are going on holiday!

On the other hand, it is not acceptable for supervisors to retain materials for lengthy periods without comment. I believe it is best for both parties to negotiate a *realistic* agreed date for return of materials when they are handed over. For a full chapter draft, a period of 2 weeks is sensible. For a full thesis draft, 4 weeks should be the minimum, depending upon the other activities of the supervisor. It should be noted that it is in both parties' interests that the supervisor(s)' comments are the result of mature and deep reflection upon the contents, not a rushed job. Saving time now can waste it at the other end of the process if major mistakes are made. Maintain some pressure but do not pester them into doing a second rate job.

STUDENT ACCESS TO RESOURCES

Most universities obtain substantial resources to support research students. While this amount does not all find its way to the department in which the student is enrolled (there are many greedy and needy intermediaries!), it is nevertheless financially worthwhile for departments to have research students on board. It is therefore appropriate that the department provides the resources necessary for the students to complete their research programmes. Most students have foregone substantial income to complete their studies and therefore do not have the resources to subsidise the university. An important role for the supervisor is to ensure that ready access to the necessary resources is achieved.

I am afraid to say that, in Australia at least, health sciences faculties do not have a good reputation for supporting their students. Some departments do not provide access to photocopying resources for their students. Others provide no office space whatsoever. It seems to me that if you are going to accept the students and the money that they generate, then it is only fair and appropriate that the basic essentials are provided for them to complete their work programmes. Such essentials in my view include:

- desk, chair and filing facilities
- access to stationery

- access to a telephone at which calls can also be received
- library access
- access to photocopying facilities (within limits)
- small-scale funds for necessary materials, reagents, etc.

Students will often seek additional support for their studies from university or external bodies, for example bursaries, scholarships or other grants. Supervisors should be available to provide referee reports and be able to boost their students' prospects in these ventures.

MANAGING STUDENT–SUPERVISOR CONFLICT

From time to time conflicts will emerge in the student–supervisor dialogue. The sources of the conflicts can be many and varied. Indeed, the source of them is largely irrelevant to how they should be managed. If there is disagreement, then the place for expression of that disagreement is directly between the participants, not with other parties. As a convenor of postgraduate studies in a busy academic department, I often had students approach me about difficulties with their supervisor(s). Before I entered into any further dialogue about the matter, I asked the student whether he or she had discussed this issue directly and fully with the supervisor(s) in order to broker a resolution. Frequently the answer was no, or only obliquely. If the answer from the student is no, I insist that the student broaches the issue directly with Dr X, no matter if it is personally embarrassing or difficult. I explain to the student that the involvement of a third party before the issue has been fully discussed is likely to inflame rather than ameliorate the situation. In these cases, when I have followed up later with the student, in almost all cases to date, the issue has been resolved to the satisfaction of the student.

However, if the student has fully discussed the issue with the supervisor(s) and the matter still has not been resolved, I then discuss the issue with the supervisor(s) in a non-emotional way. If it cannot be resolved, I then suggest to both parties that the supervisory arrangements be changed as a matter of priority. This has occurred only once in my career. I have also seen the outcomes of what has occurred when postgraduate convenors in other settings have had secret discussions with students concerning conflicts with supervisors. The usual result is an escalation of the conflict and a damaging of relationships additional to the student–supervisor relationship. The student is almost always the loser in such situations. I consider this procedure to be an ineffective and unprofessional approach to conflict management. Interestingly, it is rare that supervisors complain about their students in any sort of systematic or official way. My clear advice is, therefore, if you have conflict to deal with in your academic dialogues with the supervisor(s), do this directly. Do not involve third parties in the first instance. Of course, if the matter is an issue such as sexual harassment, by all means follow the appropriate procedures. In this instance you should be contemplating a supervisory change immediately.

MANAGING SUPERVISOR–SUPERVISOR CONFLICT

If the student has more than one supervisor, occasions can arise where they provide conflicting advice to the student. If the student meets separately with the different supervisors, as often occurs with busy schedules, this can happen inadvertently quite easily. The receipt of conflicting advice can create conflict for the student in terms of which advice should be taken.

My advice to students is that they should not attempt to resolve this issue on their own. It should be pointed out to both supervisors that they disagree and that a joint meeting is needed to discuss the issues. The student should then schedule the meeting so that all can attend. The student should wait until the meeting has been held before taking any action involving the material in conflict. I have never heard of a disagreement between supervisors that has not been resolved at a face-to-face meeting. However, if disagreement persists then the student should have one more written attempt at resolving it. If this fails, then go with the principal supervisor's advice.

3

General writing techniques and strategies

While this book deals with many specific technical details of the structure and functions of sections and chapters within the thesis, there are certain writing strategies and techniques that are applicable to all sections of the thesis. This chapter is concerned with a discussion of some of these strategies with a view to simplifying the writing process for the student. We shall first discuss the strategy of 'telling them what you are going to tell them, telling them, and telling them what you have told them'. This is followed by a discussion of the thesis plan.

TELLING THEM!

In order to improve the clarity of sections of the thesis, it is useful to employ a three-part structure when writing sections. This involves 'telling them what you are going to tell them, telling them, and telling them what you have told them'. This strategy applies to any informative piece of writing or verbal communication such as a lecture.

In the first part of the communication, you tell them what you are going to tell them. In a sentence or two, explain to the reader the content and purpose of the material that is about to follow. Something like the following text is an example of this first part of the strategy:

There has been a considerable amount of research that has investigated the association between the living arrangements of people with psychiatric disorders following discharge from hospital and readmission rates to hospital. It is proposed to review this work in the following section of the thesis.

Thus, it is clear to readers what is going to happen next. They are going to be reading about post-discharge living arrangements of people with psychiatric disorders. However, this strategy is not only applicable to the thesis literature review: it can be used throughout the thesis. For example, in the results section, something like the following could be included:

Analyses concerning the demographic characteristics of the sample participants will be presented first, followed by comparisons of these characteristics with other similar studies.

The second component of the strategy involves 'telling them'. The main information that is to be conveyed in this section of the thesis is presented next. This material could be quite voluminous. For example, with the review of post-discharge accommodation for people with psychiatric disorders, this could run to quite a few pages if a comprehensive review was presented. It is not necessary to present details of this information here for the purposes of illustration. The methods of presenting a literature review are discussed in Chapter 5.

In the third part of the presentation strategy, you tell them what you have told them. The bottom line, the point, the summary – whatever you want to call it – is conveyed here. It might go something like this:

Thus the US research has indicated that people with psychiatric disorders who live outside the family home have two to three times the rates of readmission to hospital than people who are living in the home. This has important implications for the planning of accommodation with psychiatric disorders. It also raises questions as to why the rates are so high for other living arrangements.

Or in the case of the results, it might be something like this:

We have see that the analyses of the demographic data revealed the participant group to be different from the rest of the community in several key respects. Women were over-represented as were people from ethnic minorities, especially from non-English speaking backgrounds.

Thus as a general writing strategy, the 'tell them what you are going to tell them, tell them, and tell them what you have told them' approach can improve the clarity of your writing. Sometimes these are called signposts. Signposts serve the function of telling you where you are and where you are about to go. They are very useful in theses as well as in other avenues of life!

THE IMPORTANCE OF THE THESIS PLAN

It has been previously noted that a thesis is generally a very long document, indeed the longest document you may ever write. In building terms it is a two storey house with four bathrooms. However, most builders can build this structure in a much shorter time than it takes the research student to write their thesis! A builder would not contemplate even turning the first sod without a detailed plan. Yet some students attempt to write their entire thesis without one. To put it plainly, you are going to waste a lot of time and materials if you do not have even a rudimentary plan for your thesis.

The first stage in the development of the plan is recognition of the basic thesis structure. It is not proposed to repeat this detail here, but details of the usual structure of a thesis are provided in Chapters 1 and 12. There is not a great deal of room to move in the basic thesis structure. It is pretty much universal. This structure is the plan skeleton but more detail is needed. I use plans in almost all of my writing ventures except short letters. I used the following plan to write an introduction to a short journal article on transplantation decisions that I wrote recently:

- Present some historical stuff about transplantation technology.
- Discuss how many people have transplants in different countries.
- Discuss international practices in allocation of organs to recipients.
- Discuss the problems arising from organ shortages.
- Mention xenografts and dismiss them.
- Then focus on local organ allocation procedures.
- Review current research concerning transplantation decisions at team level.
- Discuss concept of 'social worth'.
- Discuss measurement of 'social worth'.
- Since public money is used to do transplants, discuss necessity for accountability to justify research. Introduce Lichtenstein's concept of societal decision makers.
- Specify knowledge gaps in literature.
- State research questions.

Naturally, the plan for a thesis is longer because of the greater volume and scope of material, but the elements are the same. It is not necessary to plan the entire thesis in full before the commencement of writing, but you certainly need at least a basic plan for the section that you are currently writing. I find it much easier to switch around the order and scope of arguments in my plan before I start writing rather than to do this after the words are on the page or screen. In fact I spend quite a bit of time playing with my writing plans to check the scope and sequence of them. I think it is a very good idea to discuss the scope and content of a section of a thesis with the supervisor in the form of a plan prior to writing. As with building, the erasure of a line on a plan is a much simpler exercise than demolishing a just-built wall!

I also use my writing plans to guide my literature search rather than vice versa. If I am writing a paper on transplantation, then I know that I will need some papers on the history of transplantation. I go looking for them. Literature searching and the production of a review is not a passive serendipitous process. It is driven in part by your plan, i.e. what you want to say.

THESIS DRAFTS

The advent of word processors has delivered many advantages to their users. But in the wrong hands, in my opinion, they can also dramatically increase the effort required to produce the final written thesis. This is because they make it possible to bypass the drafting procedures that were forced upon academics when the process of writing was exclusively manual.

Under a manual writing process, the academic would write a first draft of the materials in full and in longhand. At the end of the first draft, the materials would be edited by reading them in full and then changes would be made on the manuscript. The paper would then be typewritten and minor edits conducted on the typewritten version. The sheer effort involved in editing written work meant that there was a strong imperative to get it right first time, or near to the first time! The wrath of the secretary on the third draft of a long typewritten text was too awful to contemplate and it was only the most thick-skinned academic who would attempt it. (Incidentally this is not some pathetic attempt on my part to recreate past glories. It is a fact that the writing process has been changed irrevocably by the invention and widespread dissemination of word processors.)

With word processors, the sequential process of drafting can be bypassed. The text presented as a draft may have already had eight passes through by the author if he or she is doing the word processing, which is usual for students. Sections may have been switched in position four times. I have even had a student present Draft version A and Draft version B, with material presented in different sequence to see which one I liked better! This would and could not have happened in the manual days. The student would have broken down from the sheer effort of producing the text.

The ability to move material around at will, insert new material and delete material is a wonderful liberation, but it can lead to great inefficiency with a nervous and/or disorganised author. Being able to think, 'Oh, I can fix that later' is not helpful to such a person.

I advocate the production of a plan for the section in question and then completion of a full draft of that section of the plan before any editing takes place. I like to leave at least a day or so between drafts so that each can be read afresh. The longer this gap the better, in terms of freshness of approach to reading the material. It is noted in the chapters concerned with the introduction and literature review (Chapter 5) and the results and discussion sections of the thesis (Chapter 9) that I advocate a layered approach to the writing of these sections, in any event. Broadly, the first pass through the material presents the factual material, the second pass involves the production of the evaluative and critical material and the third pass involves the production of the integrating material. I have found this layered approach to be very useful in breaking down what might seem to be an insurmountable task into manageable chunks. It is best performed with a rest in between layers.

A common question that arises from students is how many drafts of the thesis will be required before it is ready for submission? This is a very difficult question to answer, as it depends upon the starting quality. With my own students I generally see each thesis chapter through two drafts on its own as an individual component. When the thesis is in draft form as an entire document, this generally also takes one to two drafts to finalise. The components need to be dovetailed with each other, even when written to a closely structured plan. So, any one section would be seen three to four times by me before the thesis is finalised and submitted. Different students and supervisors have their own needs and practices.

DEALING WITH WRITER'S BLOCK

I have met very few people who genuinely like writing for its own sake. Most people like what writing does for them, i.e. to allow them to gain a degree and to be able to deposit the cheque. The process itself can be quite painful and tedious. Whoever coined the phrase 'the tyranny of the blank page' was absolutely on the mark as far I am concerned.

I do not like writing because it gives me back ache and head ache, but I very much like what it brings for me. My love of the outcomes overcomes my hatred of the process. In writing this text, I have dillied, dallied, started twice, mucked around for about 3 years on my weekends – and then I wrote it in about 3 months. Much thesis writing is the same, although it should not be. The fits and starts approach is too erratic when the result needs to be guaranteed.

Writer's block occurs when the author does not know what to do next. The contemplation of the Everest peak of a completed thesis from the base camp can fill the prospective climber with awe and trepidation. Which path should be taken? In order to overcome writer's block, a content plan is sorely needed. If there is difficulty in producing the plan, then seek the advice of your supervisor(s) to produce it. Having produced the plan, then select which part of it you are going to write. It does not matter if it is the easiest or your favourite bit. You should then follow the layered approach to writing that I have suggested in Chapters 5 and 9. It is not difficult, in a literature review for example, to write a descriptive precis of an article. From this small building block elaborate structures easily grow. If you attempt to write your thesis in one section without a plan you are setting yourself up for failure. A long journey consists of many small steps in the same direction. I think some students imagine that they are Mozart, who reputedly could produce final scores out of his head direct onto the paper. I have never met anyone who could write an academic work in this fashion, so you need to be realistic about the process. Drafting and re-drafting will be required.

THE WRITING ENVIRONMENT AND TOOLS

I cannot write at my usual work desk during work hours to save myself. The telephone rings constantly, students come to see me, colleagues drop in. I am not even safe in the library: 'Oh Dr Thomas, I called by to see you at your office but you weren't there and I thought I might find you here'. I cannot write with interruption. It takes me 10 minutes to focus on what I am supposed to be doing following the last interruption. If you are like me, to write you need no interruptions, your writing tools and resources and the desire to write, or at least the desire to finish the task for which you need to do the writing. I like to write in my study because it is quiet and I have all my stuff there. As a student, when I was less well known and pursued, I used to write in the library because everyone else had to shut up or they were thrown out! Also, most of what I needed was there in terms of research sources, dictionaries, etc. This was in the quill days when word processors were not readily available (or actually invented yet!). It is important to have a quiet place where you can do your writing.

Your co-residents need to be trained to leave you alone for periods at a time. I write in about 45-minute bursts with sticky bun rewards in between. You should devise your own rewards. People vary of course in their concentration spans, but my suggestion is that three short efficient bursts achieve more than one long burst. Also you can pretend to be actually interacting with your friends and family in between. It is hard to write when your family wants you to come out and play, so remember to play with them from time to time. If you are in trouble for not playing, tell them that you will be able to play sooner if they leave you alone.

WHAT TO WRITE WITH

I suggest a fountain pen followed by a word processor. I never write my plan or drafts first using a word processor. I like the high-speed random access provided by sheets of paper as well as the arbitrarily large amounts of memory (just add an extra few thousand sheets if more memory is required). Also one can play with paper in any sitting or lying (or eating) position. I also edit my drafts when word processed entirely on the paper copy. I never do this directly on the screen. When I have performed my edits and have a revised word processed copy, I throw the old ones away, so that I only ever have one working copy of the document. Each to their own. Find out what works for you and stick to it.

DOCUMENT SAFETY

Computers are wonderful devices but they do fail from time to time, like any appliance. It is imperative that you have adequate backup (paper and electronic) of your thesis materials at two locations so that if there is a fire or an accident, the work is not lost. Whenever I edit a document, I routinely back it up onto a floppy disk, or now I even burn CD-ROMs since the technology has become so cheap. Incidentally, do not use the same floppy disk for the whole of your candidature! Floppy disks routinely fail. Every few months create new ones and archive or throw away the old ones.

As an exercise, I recommend that you open up the case of a floppy disk and see how frail it is. Then ponder why you would risk a year's work by only having one copy on such a tiny piece of plastic. Always have up-to-date paper copies as well. If the worst comes to the worst, these can be rescanned using an optical character recognition programme with a scanner.

Another little hint. You know those paper things they put in with the diskettes? They are called labels. Whenever I mention the utility of labels in avoiding manual search through three dozen identically unlabelled disks, my graduate classes shift uneasily in their seats. It seems that the world is full of closet non-labellers. Put the labels on, with writing on them, explaining what portions of your stuff are on them! Remember that a floppy disk is a disposable item. You do not want your thesis to be disposable until you finish the examination.

THE PSYCHOLOGY OF THESIS WRITING

Writing a thesis is a creative task. It is hard to be creative when you are expecting the sheriff or the bailiffs to repossess your furniture or if you are contemplating your divorce. You may have heard of the Holmes and Rahe research concerning stressful life events in which certain events, e.g. one's own death, divorce and so on, are assigned numerical scores (Holmes & Rahe, 1967). Without a doubt writing a research thesis would receive a high stressful event score. However, this is not my point. To do any creative activity such as writing a thesis, you need a calm life and a still mind. My advice is to get your job change or divorce over and done with before you commence studying! However, if the tortured genius model suits you best, good luck with it. I think it is hard to be creative when psychologically your socks are on fire. There is another aspect of psychology and thesis writing that I think is very important, and this is having buddies who will help you share the experience and support you during it. I think the 'buddy factor' is one of the reasons why there is a moderate sized positive correlation between completion rates and the numbers of students enrolled in the departments in the study of completion rates at the University of California at San Diego previously discussed. Having other students around who are experiencing the same things you are experiencing (and hopefully culminating in successful completion of their theses) can be highly validating and motivating. Of course, your supervisor should also be a source of motivation and energy, but other students are a particularly important source of psychological support. Find a buddy or buddies and form a support group. I attribute the high completion rates of my own students to them being buddies with each other. Because they worked in related areas, they were also able to swap resources with each other and their supervisor.

The above suggestions should help you with the management of your writing and your desire to do it. Remember that, although you will eventually have to produce a very large document for your thesis, if you segment it into smaller sections and follow the procedures outlined in this text, it will happen. Choose small chunks and chew them well.

4

Determining the scope of the research programme and thesis

In designing the research programme and producing the thesis that reports it, the student has to make a number of decisions. How large should the thesis be? How much work is required to meet the requirements of the degree? While some broad guidelines are sometimes provided about thesis size, degree regulations rarely specify any details at all about the acceptable scope of the research programme. The present section deals with these issues.

My first practical suggestion for students who are in doubt about the required scope of the research programme for their degree is systematically to peruse theses that have been successfully presented for the same degree. You will no doubt find considerable variation in the size, presentation and scope of the theses. I rarely have more than half the copies of the theses of students I have supervised in my office because current students are giving them a good looking over in terms of these parameters. I suggest a thorough examination of as many theses as you can readily find. If you happen to know how the examination went as well, even better, because you can study the differences between those that went through with highly positive commendations versus those that had some difficulties (although this probably reflects idiosyncrasies among the examiners just as much as thesis quality).

THESIS SIZE

Most degree regulations specify generally the maximum overall length of the thesis required. It is important that you consult these at your host institution as a matter of priority. For Honours programmes in many universities, the thesis size may be between 10 000 and 15 000 words (40 and 60 pages of text on double-spaced pages). For coursework minor theses, a slightly larger thesis than this is generally specified. For Masters by research theses, the figure may be between 30 000 and 40 000 words (120 and 160 double-spaced pages), and for a PhD, most universities have an absolute limit of 100 000 words (400 double-spaced pages!), with a desired size of between 50 000 and 65 000 words (200 and 260 double-spaced pages). Remember, these are *maximum* sizes, not minimum.

Quite often, the stated size suggestions and regulations are not observed, and in my experience, there has been a trend towards larger theses over the last 2 decades. Perhaps this is why the research on thesis completion rates shows a commensurate lengthening in candidature times. The submission of a thesis outside these boundaries risks adverse comment. At the lower limits, the examiner may question the amount of work that has been performed by the student. Examiners like to know that sufficient suffering has occurred. If the limits are exceeded, this increases the work requirement of the examiner and he or she may question the tightness of the written text. Most students tend to worry about criticisms of insufficient scope more than they worry about the examiner's increased workload.

In my own thesis examinations, I have often found the very large theses to be quite flabbily written rather than of superior scope. Generally, they contain too much tutorial level material and unnecessary detail that would be best deleted. However, theses that contain extensive qualitative material also tend to be on the large side because of the inclusion of textual material from interview transcripts and, despite being large, can be quite tightly written. Remember to study successful examples so that the local expectations are observed by you.

Thesis scope is a more vexed issue. I am not going to make some salacious remark about size not being important, however, where theses are concerned, it does matter and furthermore, in the case of research theses, it is much more an issue of quality than quantity once within the prescribed size ranges.

RESEARCH PROGRAMME SCOPE

Several factors impact upon the requisite scope of a research programme and the thesis that is written to report it. The level of the degree for which the thesis is being presented, of course, has a large impact upon the acceptable scope of the research programme. Also, theses with a qualitative orientation have different requirements from those with a quantitative orientation.

To take quantitative empirical research projects and theses first, it is usual that an honours level or minor thesis for a masters by coursework would have one empirical study only or perhaps use secondary sources such as documents and/or previously collected data. For example, the study might be a clinical study of a small group of patients, or perhaps a social survey of a larger group of patients. Mind you, the results need to be statistically meaningful so there does need to be a decent sample size to avoid adverse examiner comment. In a social survey using an easily administered questionnaire, the expectation might be for over 100 participants in the research, depending upon the specific power requirements of the analyses to be performed. In a clinical study, perhaps a two-group intervention study with, say, a minimum of a dozen or so participants per group would be a basic expectation. However, if the measures taken contain a lot of error then the power of the design is likely to be inadequate.

In a Masters by research, if there is one study only, then it needs to be fairly decent in scope. For example, a national sample survey of professionals might suffice. In a clinical study, the sample size would need to meet the rigorous statistical power criteria expected of such research. This might be 20–30 participants per intervention or control group. Occasionally, a Masters by research will include multiple studies, particularly if the individual studies are small and easily performed. Since the Masters by research is a full research degree, the expectations with respect to scope are higher than for an Honours or minor thesis Masters. I personally think that a Masters by research is often a poor investment because the scope expectations are often similar to those of a PhD.

For a PhD, in an empirical context, it is uncommon to have a single study as the basis for the research programme. However, if it is a large-scale study with several different facets then this can be acceptable. It is much more usual to have multiple studies in the PhD research programme. Some theses I have seen have contained up to 8 such studies, but 2 or 3 studies or substantive components of the 1 study would be the norm for a health sciences PhD. The days of the single study PhD seem to be over.

For qualitative research work, the rules are much less obvious. I have seen a full Masters by research where the sole data collection comprised one-off interviews with 8 people who had experienced a particular disease. The interviews were not heavily described or intensively analysed. One of the examiners questioned the scope of the research programme but then recommended that the thesis be passed. The other examiner made no comment. I must say that I was very surprised that such a modest venture had satisfied the examiners. Had I been examining the thesis, I would have probably requested more work from the student because of insufficient programme and thesis scope. If the research participants had been drawn from a very rare group of people (for example, recent English prime ministers), then perhaps this might have balanced the very small numbers. However, in this instance the condition was a high prevalence one and the 8 had been chosen in a reasonably biased fashion.

I make these remarks from the perspective of a researcher who routinely performs both qualitative and quantitative research. Eight interviews for a Masters, whether in depth or shallow, is an absolute holiday. It would have some difficulty making it for a journal article in many journals in the field. I do not believe that performing qualitative research work releases investigators from the basic requirement of demonstrating that their research findings are generalisable to and useful for others with the same predicaments, no matter how good the theoretical sampling. For students who are performing qualitative work for their thesis research programme, I would suggest a minimum of 20 participants for a Masters by research and 2 similar-sized studies as the minimum for a PhD.

With my own students for the PhD, I routinely advocate the use of a mixed method strategy, i.e. the inclusion of both qualitative and quantitative studies in the thesis. My rationale for this approach is the heartfelt conviction that both methodological approaches have inherent strengths and weaknesses that are complementary (see Polgar & Thomas, 1995, for a discussion of these issues). I advocate a methodological triangulation in order to maximise the validity and robustness of the findings in the research programme. To date this approach has been well received by examiners.

Of course not all theses are empirical in nature, although most in the health sciences employ data collection methods of one form or another. For non-empirical theses such as historical analyses, where the data collection involves purely documentary sources, the picture as to appropriate scope is even less clear. I have no advice other than to consult with experts in the disciplinary area in which you are working. While the use of multidisciplinary approaches to knotty research problems is now frequently advocated in research in general, I think that doing a thesis in which there are no obvious examiners with the same knowledge base and epistemological and methodological base is a risk.

The scope of the thesis and research programme is also not simply defined by the size of the data collection endeavour in the thesis. The literature review and analysis in a thesis stand alone from any empirical component. In an Honours thesis, a good 15–20 pages of literature review precedes any empirical reporting and analysis. In Masters by coursework theses, the expectation might be for 20–30 pages of such material. In Masters by research and PhD theses, the expectation might be for 30–40 pages of such material. Reviews substantially below or above these figures, in my experience, may incur the wrath of the examiners in terms of insufficient scope or insufficient focus. It is difficult to prescribe the exact length of these components because they are determined by the individual research programme, but I have based my estimates on quite a few years of close observation of what seems to be acceptable to other thesis examiners.

Thus while thesis size is a fairly routine if variable parameter, the scope of the research programme is more vexed. Students are encouraged to study closely theses passed at their institution for the same degree for which they are studying with a view to determining acceptable scope.

5

The introduction and literature review

Before discussing the production of the introduction and literature review, it is necessary to consider the overall chapter structure of the thesis. In some theses, the introduction is presented as a stand-alone chapter involving a short statement of intent followed by a detailed literature review chapter. Sometimes there are even two literature review chapters with different areas of literature presented in each of the chapters.

I do not favour this type of structure because it assumes that the rationale for the thesis and setting the scene can be presented separately from the literature review. I find this to be a strange proposition since the scene that is being set is significantly dependent upon a discussion of the findings of previous work in the area. There is no requirement for chapters in the thesis to be of equal length, which might be behind the reasoning for some of the thesis structures I have encountered. In a sense the abstract has already provided the reader with an overview of what is to come, so I do not see the need for a stand-alone, essentially literature-free, chapter to do this.

I favour a large single introductory chapter in which the rationale for the thesis, the historical context and the previous relevant research are presented as one integrated whole. Of course, if the student or supervisor favours a different structure, then that should be pursued. It is most unlikely that this will attract adverse comment from the examiners unless it is a particularly bizarre arrangement.

THE FUNCTIONS OF THE THESIS INTRODUCTION

Essentially the introduction to a health sciences thesis ought to perform the following functions in the thesis document:

1. provide a rationale for the thesis research
2. review current knowledge in the fields relevant to the thesis through the performance of a literature review and analysis

3. culminate in the statement of the research questions to be answered by the work in the thesis.

It is now proposed to discuss each of these functions in turn.

DEVELOPING THE THESIS RATIONALE

An important function of the introduction is to provide a rationale for the thesis research. The thesis rationale is concerned with answering the question 'Why does this work need to be done?' While you might be convinced that your thesis topic is of obvious and intrinsic merit, it is the views of the examiners that count! Therefore it is important that you are able to communicate effectively to them a plausible and convincing rationale for the work you have performed and which you are attempting to report in the thesis.

The rationale for the thesis is not confined to any one section of the thesis, but it ought be particularly concentrated throughout the introductory chapter. It needs to be woven closely into the fabric of the introduction and literature review.

A number of standard arguments can be used to defend the research work included in your thesis and can be used in the development of your rationale. These arguments are discussed below in plain English form.

This is something we do not know already

The most basic rationale for studying something is that we do not know about it already. If we did know it already, then why would we bother to research it? If you wish to use a bit of jargon, we could say the thesis introduction has to identify clearly the 'knowledge gaps' that need to be filled. The knowledge gap rationale is a bit weak on its own (i.e. we do not know this so we should), but it is a basic requisite for the other possible arguments in the rationale to be made. The knowledge gap argument is a kind of Sir Edmund Hilary 'because it is there' explanation of why we need to know. An example of some text that expresses this type of argument follows:

Thus the literature review has revealed that the state of knowledge in the literature is unsatisfactory concerning whether long-term survivors of HIV (as defined by 10 years following infection without progression to AIDS) have psychological characteristics that are different from those who have not survived. Accordingly, the research programme was designed to examine this proposition.

Other people think this problem is important

A second line of argument for a thesis programme rationale is that other people think the problem is important too. This relies on finding people who have said that your general research agenda or approach is worth pursuing. Once again, this is not a particularly compelling stand-alone rationale as it is a sort of appeal to authority or adherence to academic group norms. All the in-crowd wear dungarees and hang around at the local coffee shop, so we should do this as well.

On the basis of these results, Temoshok (1988) asserted that 'a biopsychosocial approach to AIDS research is necessary and ... may provide critical information for understanding and treating AIDS' (p. 188)

The above quotation is an excerpt from a paper that I wrote recently concerning the psychological characteristics of people with HIV who have survived their illness for a long time. I was arguing, as a psychologist, that psychological constructs had not been included in the studies of long-term survival because the medical researchers had advocated totally biomedical cellular level explanations for health hardiness. I went on to cite evidence for the existence of direct links between psychological states and immune competence in humans. One of my arguments along the way was that people like Temoshok were supporting the approach I was advocating. Thus I was using Temoshok as an appeal to authority justification for studying what I was studying, i.e. we were wearing the same colour dungarees.

The problem I am studying affects lots of people in a particularly unfortunate way and/or costs a lot of money

Now we are talking! This aspect of the rationale is often fairly easy to develop in health science theses. If you are studying people with a particular health problem, then a presentation of the epidemiology of that problem is de rigueur. Even better, if it costs the community a lot of money. You can include statements about the fabulous cost of the condition and how, if your research bears fruit, this fabulous cost could be reduced. The following excerpt from one of my papers on back pain does the trick:

For some time, back injuries have attracted considerable research attention across a wide range of countries. In Sweden, Andersson (1979) reported that 'back sickness' accounted for on average 12.5% of the days lost due to occupational injury among Swedish workers. In the UK, Anderson (1981) estimated that 7.3% of the total sick days were due to low back pain, representing a loss of 15 million work days per annum. David (1985), however, reported that sprains and strains to the back at work, in the UK, accounted for an average of 14.9% of all work absences over 3 days for the period 1978 to 1980, representing approximately 250 000 cases for each year. Benn & Wood (1975) estimated that 13 000 000 visits per annum to general practitioners in the UK were associated with low back problems and that there were 6000 low back operations each year.

So why are you not out there studying back injuries? The point I was establishing was that this is a high-prevalence costly condition that requires study because of the issues. Later on in this paper, I went into how much it all costs. This is not a particularly academically respectable argument but it certainly gets the community's attention. Most theses can stand a dose of this sort of epidemiological contextualisation of the work reported within it.

Solving this problem has implications for other problems

It can be argued that solutions to problems within a particular field may have wider implications. For example, the discovery of a vaccine for a particular virus may lead to the use of similar techniques for other viruses. If I were performing a study of the health problems of nurses arising from shiftwork, I might feel moved to write something like this:

While the particular occupational group chosen for inclusion within the present research was nurses, there is no reason to suppose that the findings would not be generalisable to all health workers involved in regular shiftwork.

In animal work, the anthropomorphic argument is a form of this argument.

The liver function of the pig has been found to be a particularly useful model of human liver function in that...

The research is theoretically important and interesting

If the research involves the test of a particular theoretical approach to understanding the research problem, then it can be argued that the work has important theoretical implications. Although the other arguments presented above are useful arguments to include in a discussion of thesis topic rationale, the theoretically important line of argument is probably the most academically respectable. Some words that might express this line of argument follow:

Thus the proposed research will provide a direct test of the cross-cultural validity of the Health Belief Model in explaining health care service utilisation by people from Australian Greek and Australian Anglo-Celtic backgrounds. The validity of the model has important implications for the prediction and understanding of the utilisation of services.

It will enable us to do it better

Health scientists often have a strongly applied orientation and therefore warm to the discussion of practice implications of any research. Claims that interventions may be better targeted, more effective, more efficient, cost less, etc., as a result of the research, are also certain to put a partial smile on the examiners' faces. This is because the researcher has taken the effort to connect his or her work to the context in which it is performed as well as, perhaps, striven to make the world a slightly better place.

There are, of course, many other possible lines of argument that can be advanced to support the conduct of a research programme. However, the above lines of argument are frequently employed in the construction of the rationale for research theses and all ought be considered for inclusion in the rationale.

HOW TO WRITE A LITERATURE REVIEW

One of the areas of the thesis in which many students struggle is the production of the literature review. I consider that this is because they try to adopt the Mozartian approach of writing it all in one pass and in one sitting. I have developed a method of writing reviews that I have found to be very effective and efficient. Before we discuss this approach, let us consider the function of a review.

A literature review has several functions. The most important of these are that it should:

1. review current knowledge in fields relevant to the thesis
2. describe the characteristics of previous studies in the area, including who conducted them, where they were conducted, who were the participants, what protocols were followed and what were the findings and conclusions

3. compare and contrast relevant studies and findings
4. comment on the strengths and limitations of the relevant studies and findings
5. identify any gaps in knowledge pertinent to the research questions to be addressed by the thesis.

A literature review should be *informative*, *evaluative* and *integrative*. These attributes correspond to the three stages that I advocate in the construction of a literature review. I suggest that students first write the informative detail of the studies to be reviewed in a neutral way. I suggest they then add critical (this does not always mean negative) analysis of the literature they have just described. They should then integrate the various studies to compare and contrast their findings. All three elements (information, evaluation and integration) are needed to produce a high-quality literature review.

When I write a literature review I take all the studies I think I might include in my review and neutrally describe what happened within the studies. I try to answer the questions 'who?', 'what?', 'where?' and 'when?' for each of the studies I am going to highlight in the review. After having written these informative but neutral and separate mini-abstracts of each article, I then draft the critical and integrating materials. These additions make an enormous difference to the quality of the review. Let us now turn to specific examples of how the descriptive, evaluative and integrative layers are constructed in a literature review.

Consider the following examples of descriptions of a study:

1. Thomas, Stone & Greenwood (1990) found that age and length of compensation insurance claim were correlated in injured workers.
2. Thomas, Stone & Greenwood (1990) performed an epidemiological analysis of 65 000 compensation insurance claims for injured workers in the Australian state of Victoria in 1989. They found a correlation of +0.98 between the age of the worker and the average length of time spent by the worker on compensation insurance benefits. This suggests that older workers may take longer to recover, when injured, than do younger workers.

Example (1) above may be satisfactory for an abbreviated summary or a short journal article or if it is part of a very minor point. However, for a research thesis, it is simply not adequate. Example (2) provides the bare bones description of the study being reviewed. It also indicates that the reviewer has probably read the paper! This is the type of mini-abstract or study description that I write first when I am constructing my literature review. However, even the detailed study description provided in (2) above still lacks an evaluative comment. That is, the study is described neutrally without any evaluation of whether the study was sound or not. We do not know whether we should accept the findings of the study as their validity is not evaluated.

This *evaluative* material is what I write in the next layer of the literature review. Suitable examples of such critique that could be added might include:

Thomas et al's study is, in fact, a population study as the jurisdiction they studied had compulsory notification of all worker's compensation claims at that time. Therefore, the trends discovered are likely to be robust since they were based on a population study of 65 000 claims.

or alternatively:

The analysis conducted in Thomas et al's study could be criticised on the grounds that individual case data were not available to the researchers owing to confidentiality considerations. They were, therefore, unable to partial out the effects of other extraneous variables in their analyses.

Thus we now have a full description of the study and a statement about whether it is any good or not.

The next step is to *integrate* this material with other studies. We know what Thomas et al think. But what do other researchers in the field think? These guys might be crazy and no-one else might agree with them. Let us examine what might be written to assist with this integration of material with other work in the field.

Thomas et al's findings are consistent with those of Whacklow, Furtle & Crun (1989). In their study of 2000 workers' compensation claims in a large county of Ireland, Whacklow et al also found a strong association between age and claim duration. However, the study by Dunn (1989) conducted in Chicago with US workers found no such association.

These additional statements integrate the current state of knowledge with other studies.

Incidentally, each article does not need the full treatment as given above. If you did this for every article you included, you would write a very long review and bore the reader something ferocious. Give the key articles the full treatment as above, but the others can be described more economically. However, beware of long lists of references with no evaluative or integrative input. This is not likely to please your examiners. They want to know that you have the expertise to be discriminating.

You can include critique and evaluation with a word: celebrated, oft-cited, flawed, seminal, excellent, authoritative and so on. However, whenever I use single word critique, my co-authors edit out my single word epithets and awards. This is why I have written this book on my own!

EVALUATION AND CRITIQUE

It is important to maintain balance in the literature review. If there are features of the studies and work to criticise, then by all means do so. However, if you read your review and discover that, according to you, every study cited includes major mistakes except your own work, you have probably overdone the negativity of the review. This uniform negativity may also not be readily accepted by examiners who are experts working in the field(s) you are reviewing, as they are likely to have published within it! You may be implicitly or explicitly calling them numbskulls. Highly enjoyable I am sure if you like the return treatment in your examination.

On the other hand, do not be afraid. If, according to your literature review, no one has made any mistakes, you have not been sufficiently critical in your review. You have produced a literature list not a review. The reader may just as well read the article abstracts instead of your 'review'. Think of how a theatre critic writes a review. First the plot is described factually, then the strengths and weaknesses are discussed, then the critic reaches some conclusions. You should follow this model in your thesis literature review. I should say that I have read many examination reports where the examiner has said something like 'the student has merely provided a list of some of the relevant literature; there is insufficient critique'. I cannot recall reading a report where the examiner has been stung by the level of criticism in a review.

SIZE OF THE INTRODUCTORY CHAPTER

Naturally this is a function of the level of research degree and hence the ultimate size of the thesis. As discussed in Chapter 4, Honours theses may total between 10 000 and 15 000 words with

Masters by research theses normally totalling about 30 000–40 000 words, while for a PhD the total size is normally between about 50 000 and 65 000 words, depending upon the discipline and the local rules. In an Honours thesis, the proportion of that total allocated to the introduction and literature review is usually greater than for other degrees. There are limits to how small an introduction and review can be before the scope and quality are compromised. Typically, in an Honours thesis an introduction and literature review chapter runs to between 15 and 20 pages (3500–5000 words). In a Masters thesis the corresponding figure is about 20 to 30 pages (5000–7500 words), and for a PhD between 30 and 40 pages (7500–10 000 words) is typical.

If the introduction is significantly shorter or longer than the suggested ranges, then this may attract adverse comment from the examiners. Two important features of a quality literature review are good scope and focus. Of course, in extraordinary circumstances, there may be justification for an especially short or long introduction and review. Just be prepared for the 'lack of focus and interminable length' or 'insufficient coverage of the relevant literature' comments in the examiners' reports if the introduction is excessively long or short.

Some research student literature reviews include little description of the studies, combined with a lot of critique. Thus the review may be long on rhetoric and short on facts. Sometimes the opposite problem occurs where much description is given of the research studies, but little critique and integration is provided. Thus, the literature review needs to have strong informative, evaluative and integrative components to it.

SELECTION OF LITERATURE FOR INCLUSION IN THE LITERATURE REVIEW

Part of the skill in constructing a literature review is the ability to make connections between relevant materials and to choose which information to include and which information to omit.

Reading other literature reviews in the same area is a useful guide to these decisions. For example, if a particular study or theory is routinely discussed in similar material, it is a reasonable expectation of the examiners that you will at least acknowledge the primacy of this work by discussing it in your own review. This does not mean that you have to agree with it, but you definitely should discuss it in order to demonstrate that you know of the work and its impact upon the field.

As discussed in Chapter 6, the thoroughness with which the literature-searching process is performed is the best insurance for ensuring that all previous work relevant to your thesis is found. In Chapter 6, the strategies that ought be employed in the search process are described at length. A further source of assistance in your decisions as to inclusion or exclusion of material in your literature review is your supervisor(s). As experienced authors and experts in the field they will be well placed to give you advice about the scope of your review.

However, experience need not inoculate you against errors in these decisions. I remember vividly obtaining a review of a paper I had written on a study that had employed a theory called Social Judgement Theory. The reviewer noted that I had not included reference to work by an eminent researcher, Berndt Brehmer. He or she noted that an article about Social Judgement Theory without reference to the work of Brehmer was like reading the Bible without reference to Moses! The reviewer was absolutely correct on this point, if somewhat extravagant in the choice of language. This review has certainly stuck in my mind.

THESIS AIMS AND RESEARCH QUESTIONS

It has been previously noted that one of the functions of the introduction to the thesis is to 'culminate in the statement of the research questions to be answered by the work in the thesis' and that the literature review should 'identify any gaps in knowledge pertinent to the research questions to be addressed by the thesis'. These are both different sides of the same coin. The literature review needs to conclude with an explicit summary statement of 'what we know' and 'what we do not' in order that the research questions can develop from the review.

It is imperative that the thesis has clear and unambiguous research aims and questions. These questions need to develop logically from the literature review and be supported by the thesis rationale. The research questions are normally stated at the conclusion of the introduction and they are used over and over throughout the thesis. They form the basis for the methodology. They are the basis upon which the results are presented. Since the aim of the thesis is to pose and answer the research questions, the discussion and conclusion sections necessarily focus on them. If they are not well developed then the thesis quality can be severely compromised. It is also important that the research aims and questions do not loom out of the fog of the literature review without warning. They should develop logically from the materials reviewed.

In terms of the relationship between research aims, questions and hypotheses, consider the following example for a hypothetical quantitative study:

The aim of this research was to study the relationship between age and decision-making performance.

The research question addressed by Study 1 was: 'Is there an association between age and decision-making performance on the risk propensity measure provided by the gambling task?'.

It was hypothesised that there would be a negative association between participant age and the risk propensity score derived from the gambling task completed by the participants.

Let us now consider a qualitative example of the same sort of thing:

The aim of this research was to examine the discourses of gay men who had survived 10 years since their infection with HIV without progression to AIDS.

The research questions addressed by the interview study were: What were the recurrent themes in the discourses of the gay men? Were these themes universal across the men or were they idiosyncratic? How were the discourses and themes for the gay men similar to and different from those obtained from long-term survivors of cancer?

In qualitative research, the term hypothesis does not have the same meaning as in the quantitative domain. However, it is certainly appropriate to discuss the expectations based upon previous work and experience in the area under study.

The research aims and questions are placed at the end of the introduction. It is quite appropriate to indicate where the research questions are to be addressed in the thesis. For example:

This research question was addressed by Study 2, which involved a survey of ... This Study is described in Chapter 3 of the thesis.

This type of forward notice has been previously discussed in the 'tell them' strategy described in Chapter 3. It provides a bit of cross-bracing for the thesis structure.

I sometimes use what I call a content/method matrix where I relate the research questions to the research activities or studies I have performed in a project. It looks something like this:

Research question	Study 1	Study 2	Study 3

What I do with the matrix is to relate the research questions in the thesis to the activities that I have performed in the research programme and also in the reporting of the study outcomes, stripped of the all complex words that allow us to make big strategic mistakes. Research is about answering questions. The reader needs to know what the questions are, how you have gone about answering them and what answers you have come up with. The matrix reminds me of what the questions are and how the studies are proposed to answer them. Incidentally, empty rows and columns in this table are bad! This means that your studies do not answer your questions. Believe me, the examiners will notice. Let us now turn to how we can keep your literature under control.

6

Keeping your literature under control

There are several basic strategies and procedures for locating the literature that is pertinent to your research topic. These include computer-assisted searches using electronic databases or the Internet more generally, searches using printed collected abstracts, manual literature searching and consultations with experts in the field. It is proposed to review the mechanics and advantages and disadvantages of each.

COMPUTER-ASSISTED LITERATURE SEARCHING

Most university libraries now maintain various computer-based literature databases, often stored using CD-ROM technology. The user conducts a search by first accessing the relevant databases. Then the user keys in a combination of subject keywords and also the names of key authors in the field, in order to locate all the works they have written (at least those that appear in the database). Computerised literature databases are a superb tool but only if used skillfully. If not, it is possible to make many mistakes. There are several cautions that need to be made with the use of CD-ROM-based searches.

First, most databases cover only a short period of time. If the search is to be conducted over, say, several decades, then a fair deal of repetition is required. The 'search parameters' need to be applied over and over to the various database files that correspond to the desired time intervals. It is only small databases that usually have everything to date consolidated onto the one file because the files simply do not fit, even when using high-volume storage media such as CD-ROM.

Second, most databases rely on the user selecting keywords that correspond to the ones that the authors of the research chose to describe their work. There is considerable idiosyncrasy in the ways in which authors describe their work. So there is a good chance that, even with the use of a wide range of search keywords, you will miss key articles in your topic and search area. To guard against this problem it is desirable to use quite a range of keywords in order to conduct your search. Even so, it is worthwhile to assume that only 50% of the pertinent articles in the relevant database will be discovered by you using the search methods you have employed, if you are a new user.

It should also be noted that not all journals are necessarily scanned by the larger databases. This is especially applicable to the health sciences, where many of the journals are new, or may not be of premier quality in the eyes of the database managers. Some of the well-known indexing and abstracting services, such as the US National Library of Medicine's Medline research abstract database or Psychological Abstracts, simply may not gather information from the journals you read or need to include in the thesis. There are some health sciences-specific databases such as CINAHL that are attempting to address this problem. However, for the health scientist this means that it is prudent to search all of the major relevant databases rather than just one.

While the use of computer-based search methods has some drawbacks if not performed skilfully, there are many advantages associated with the use of these techniques. Since the information is available in electronic form, it is possible to capture your search onto a disk and to use this information in its computerised form.

This can be done in a low-technology procedure, where the user dumps the information in its Medline or other database formatted form into a word processing file and then edits all the formatting off it and strips away the gunge of extra tabs, spaces, etc. In a higher technology procedure, it is possible to use software specifically designed for the purpose to import the information directly into a literature database maintained by the student. Such databases are discussed later in this chapter. These packages have come a long way in ease of use in recent years.

The Internet is an essential resource for a researcher. There are now some wonderful resources available on the Internet. The best for medical and health sciences researchers would have to be the publicly available version of Medline, known as PubMed (at the time of writing this was available at www.ncbi.nlm.nih.gov/PubMed/but check using your favourite search engine if this address does not seem to work). PubMed is a free version of the Medline you can obtain at your local library. It has some big advantages. For a start, all the 9 million citations are on one megalithic database. No swapping of CD-ROMs is required. I also like the PubMed search engine and user interface because you can do wonderful things. For example, you can search in the journal database for journal names in the topic areas. I never fail to find journals in PubMed that I have not heard of before. I highly recommend it. For the health and medical sciences it is the definitive resource. You need to become expert in its use.

You should also consider doing broader Internet searches for materials. Many agencies have materials on the web that are extremely useful. There are Cochrane sites with reviews of very many topics, as well as sites devoted to evidence-based practice with a vast number of similar reviews (just type 'Cochrane' into your search engine and prepare for the deluge). There is an explosion of developments on the Internet occurring right now.

If you are interested in health policy and/or service provision, there is a wealth of sites on the Internet that you need to visit. Most American federal agencies have large sites and Health Canada also has a very large site. Most sites allow for their public domain documents to be downloaded typically using a product such as Adobe Acrobat, which has become a de facto standard because it is in such widespread use.

These days being a researcher requires high level Internet access and skills. You need to get on the web and surf regularly. To do this from home, you need a PC, a modem, a telephone line that is not needed for people actually to contact you, some browser software (for which Internet Explorer and Netscape Navigator have achieved almost total market domination) and an Internet Service Provider. Most universities provide dial-up connection for their students and act as the service provider for their students, but this type of access in most universities is a combination of slow and/or limited. On-campus access is generally faster because the computers are connected directly to the Internet.

SEARCHES OF COLLECTED PRINTED ABSTRACTS

This is the manual, low-technology, version of the computerised searches described above. In the reference section of the library, you will find shelves-full of books of abstracts with associated author and subject indices to guide you around them. The same caveats discussed for electronic database searches apply to this form of searching. It is also possible to subscribe to some specialised abstracting services that provide regular updates to individual users using search parameters defined by the subscriber.

MANUAL SEARCHING METHODS

This process involves hitting the library shelves. If you are early on in your literature search process, it is useful to find some text-books and read their reviews of the literature pertinent to your topic, in order to discover key works in the field. Later on, you will discover that even books published today were actually written several years ago and hence will be a little dated. You will generally not find the most up-to-date literature in a textbook. However, integrative texts can be very helpful early on in the process in developing an overview and historical perspective of the area. This will help you to locate the main authors and the main places where they publish to assist your searches later.

The basic strategy for a manual search is simple. Most libraries maintain separate lists of their journal subscriptions. Inspect this list with a view to possible interest for your research topic and locate the journals of promise. If you have already read some reviews in books, you will have compiled a list of journals in which the key authors will have published work. Having located the journal titles of interest, go to the journal stacks and start looking! For example, I might decide that *Archives of Physical Medicine and Rehabilitation* is one of the journals for me. I will go to the stacks and start with the most recent journals and go back through the years. Many students ask how far they should go back. What I do in my own searches is to go back 10 years and to rely on the integrative reviews and the literature published within the last 10 years to inform me of any crucial materials that have occurred before then.

Of course, another source of key references is your supervisor(s). The supervisor(s) should be able to provide key references in your chosen field and advise you as to the scope of your search. Ask them to nominate the key journals in the field in order that you may search them. Many supervisors will scan the literature during the course of the candidature and alert the student to any relevant publications.

Another source of immense value is a high-quality review article in your topic area. Some journals specialise in review articles only. For example, the Annual Review series (e.g. *Annual Review of Public Health, Annual Review of Psychology*) publish high-quality and integrative reviews of topics on a regular basis. Some journals specialise in state-of-the-art reviews. It is difficult to overstate the value of finding such a review. Of course, many journals also intersperse such reviews with their normal empirical paper fare. In addition, journals will occasionally run special issues in a particular topic. If this topic is yours, then you will acquire a wonderful resource. All the key players will be there, probably giving comprehensive citations of their relevant material as well as the work of many others.

CONSULTING OTHER EXPERTS

A further source of key references is other academics. If you know of any academics in the field who are accessible in person or by telephone or by email, call them up or email them and ask them if they could point you to their recent work. You could also ask them to nominate what they consider to be the most significant recent work in the field. Most academics will be flattered at the attention, especially if you are polite. When you are a fair way down the track of your search, it is also useful to write to some of the leading lights and say something like the following:

Dear Professor Bloggs,

I am a research student who is conducting research in the field of xyz. I have followed your work with interest and would appreciate it if you could forward to me copies of any recent in-press work you have performed in the area.

Yours, etc.

This way you will obtain the work that is in train at the moment, which may not appear in press for another 2 years. Also, should this person become an examiner later, he or she will have a positive view of you, a small recognition factor, and will think you are a genius for citing his or her current work!

Some research centres maintain monograph or work-in-progress series in which papers submitted for publication, in press or not submitted for publication elsewhere are show-cased. These monograph series can be an invaluable source of information.

Following your manual searches do not be surprised if you locate many materials not revealed by the computer-assisted area of your search. I find that typically more than half of the references that I finally include in the reviews that I write were not revealed by my first or second pass electronic searching. However, the electronic searches are still of immense value and can save a lot of time and energy. Just do not rely on them as your sole port of call.

SUGGESTED ORDER OF THE DIFFERENT TYPES OF SEARCHES

In terms of the order of sequence of searching, I normally pursue the following sequence.

1. Locate integrative reviews in texts.
2. Conduct an electronic search using the keywords and authors located in (1) above. Perhaps now speak to your expert(s) for advice.
3. Conduct a manual search of relevant journals.
4. Using the keywords and authors found, conduct another electronic search.
5. Start reading on a regular basis the journals where you have located most materials of relevance to you. Since your candidature, in the case of a higher degree, may last several years, you need to monitor regularly the literature and keep up to date. In fact, at the last moment before the submission of the thesis, I recommend to students that they repeat their electronic search using their usual search parameters to check that nothing new and vital has appeared.

ORGANISATION AND FILING OF LITERATURE MATERIALS

Organisation of the literature materials, if done well, can save you an enormous amount of time, and conversely, if done badly, can waste an enormous amount of time.

Notwithstanding the advantages of electronic databases, I maintain a manual system alongside my electronic system. This is what I do. When I discover a reference that I want to include in my database, I obtain a physical copy of it and I prepare a card like that shown on the next page.

Bucknall, T.K. & Thomas, S.A. (1995, in press)
Critical care nurse satisfaction with levels
of involvement in clinical decisions.
Journal of Advanced Nursing

Photocopy of abstract

On the back of the card, I write any notes that I consider to be important in my interpretation of the research findings. I go to some effort to ensure that the way in which I have entered the reference citation upon the system card is the same as the style standard I am going to use in the document I am preparing. As I have previously said, I also have this information electronically stored, generally in one of the software packages designed to handle this. So, if I need a different style standard, a few button pushes generally achieve the desired result.

The actual articles I then file in alphabetical order. I advise strongly against the filing of articles in thematic groupings. My reasons for this advice include the fact that as time unfolds you may change radically your ideas about these themes and then you have an unpleasant filing task to re-file the articles. Second, alphabetical order never fails. You will always be able to locate the article if it is filed in a consistent way. Incidentally, my stationer loves me because I file the articles in lever arch files with a separate index sheet and label.

For whole books and reports without an identifiable abstract, I still have cards, but without a photocopied abstract.

I strongly advocate the use of the above system. The ability to locate your reference materials easily is basic and essential. The above system delivers a high level of performance if you adhere to it.

THE SCOPE OF LITERATURE COLLECTIONS

The typical thesis (whatever that is) contains a fair list of reference citations. An Honours thesis might contain say 40 citations, and Masters and PhD theses might contain over 100 citations. Your article library may contain many references that you do not end up citing in your thesis. If it is many, many more than you use in the final thesis then you have wasted a lot of time and money. I know of some article libraries compiled by students that have reached four figures in size. Get a grip on reality, guys! Simply listing this volume of references would be as long as a large thesis. It is important that your thesis contains all the relevant work, but your literature collection needs to be focused and selective. It is a means to an end, not an end in itself. The examiners will never hear of the huge amount of time and money you wasted in collecting the hundreds of extra references that you did not use in your thesis!

BIBLIOGRAPHIC SOFTWARE

There is a range of excellent products that are available to assist with the maintenance of literature citations and reference lists in a computer database. Probably the most popular within the health and medical sciences settings are End-Note, Pro-Cite and Reference Manager, which incidentally are now owned by one company. Each package enables the user to key in the reference details and to produce a perfectly formatted reference list in a range of arbitrary style standards. It is very smooth indeed. Each also has an extra module that permits the capture of material from the major databases such as Medline and then its direct importation into the reference database. This obviates the need for re-typing of the reference material captured in the computer search. These are fine products and there are also others that may be available to you locally.

Bibliographic tools, like the use of the Internet, can save you a lot of time and deliver a higher quality outcome than manual methods. You need to invest time to be trained in their use and application. Attend any courses you can and get out there and play.

7

The thesis methodology

This chapter is intended to assist the student with the reporting of the thesis methodology in a manner that is likely to satisfy the thesis examiners. It is not intended to be a full-scale primer of research design, as this is beyond the scope of the present book. There are other texts that deal with these issues (see for example Polgar & Thomas, 1995; Minichiello et al, 1995). However, in health sciences theses, there are recurrent issues in the structure and reporting of the method used in the research that will be considered in the later sections of this chapter.

Methodology is an important aspect of knowledge generation. In the literature review it is important that discussion occurs of the methodological stances taken by previous researchers and that their respective strengths and weaknesses are discussed when evaluating the presented work. The methodological themes raised in the introduction should connect with those discussed in the thesis methodology section(s).

The structure of the individual thesis determines where the method section(s) are to be placed. In a single study research programme, the methodology would normally precede the (first) results chapter and would normally be a separate chapter or section, albeit one that is much shorter than, for example, the introductory chapter(s). The relative shortness of the chapter is of no significance. Thesis chapters do not have to be of equivalent lengths.

It should be noted that the method section in a journal article is quite different in scope from a methodology section in a health sciences thesis. In a journal article, because of space considerations, there is usually little or almost no defence of the methodology, except perhaps in some oblique references to the strengths and limitations of the work. The method section in a journal article contains almost no explanation or rationale for the methodological choices made. This is not an adequate strategy for the health sciences thesis. The methodological decisions taken need to be discussed and defended in a systematic and robust manner.

I advocate the use of a standard method section structure and a methodological defence irrespective of whether the research has a quantitative or qualitative focus. Both approaches involve knowledge gathering and generation based on procedures and assumptions that need to be explicated. The examiners need to be convinced that the student has an expert understanding of the strengths and weaknesses of the techniques chosen and their theoretical underpinnings. The specific methodological approach chosen in no way exempts the student from this obligation.

Further, in most health sciences theses irrespective of methodological orientation, there are human participants who need to be described, tools that were used in the research and protocols in the data gathering and analysis that were followed. In addition to the standard structure, I also advocate the addition of a section entitled 'Methodology defence or rationale', in which the student defends and provides a rationale for the protocols and procedures employed in his or her work. Let us examine the content of each component of the method section in a health sciences thesis.

RESEARCH PARTICIPANTS/SUBJECTS

This is typically a very brief section, perhaps a half double-spaced page to a page. It should describe the numbers of participants in the research and their basic attributes including age, sex and diagnostic groupings if appropriate. Describe the inclusion (and any exclusion) criteria for their participation in the research. It is sometimes useful to include a table summarising the participants' demographic attributes at this point in the thesis. An example of the sort of detail required follows.

42 volunteers participated in the present research. There were 22 men and 20 women with a mean age of 53.2 years. The participants' demographic characteristics are summarised in Table 1. Participants were all current rheumatoid arthritis patients at the Rheumatology Institute who attended in the month of February, 1999. Of the 60 people approached for recruitment into the study, 42 agreed, yielding a response rate of 70%.

It is compulsory that the age and sex characteristics of the research participants are described. It is also essential that the response rate, i.e. the percentage of people who were approached to participate in the study, and who actually participated, is disclosed. This is an essential piece of information. It requires that good records are kept concerning who was approached and who finally participated. If this information is not provided then the reader has no indication of how representative the participants might be of those who could have participated in the study. This issue also needs to be taken up in the strengths and limitations of the present research section of the conclusions chapter (see Chapter 10).

RESEARCH TOOLS

This section should describe the use of any research instruments or tools employed by the researcher in the conduct of his or her research. In laboratory research, this section is labelled 'Apparatus'. As these research tools are introduced they should be reviewed and defended. That is, not only should the tools used be described, but also the reasons for their selection. This section could run for several pages in a higher degree thesis. It should be shorter for an Honours thesis.

Some example excerpts for such defences follows:

The Spielberger State Trait Anxiety Inventory (STAI) was employed to assess the participants' anxiety levels during the research programme. The Inventory provides two scores: the state score, which measures the participant's anxiety at the particular moment, and the trait score, which measures their general propensity for anxiousness. The Spielberger is a psychometrically sound instrument. Studies of its concurrent validity (see, for example, Bloggs, 1993) and test–retest reliability (see, for example, Nurk, 1994) show consistently high coefficients (0.8 to 0.95) Fotheringham's (1994) review of anxiety measurement instruments also supported the use of the Spielberger with community groups. The STAI has been used in several hundred published studies (Fotheringham, 1994).

Where the tools are not standardised and/or well known, then they need to be described in detail so that the reader understands exactly what has occurred.

Each of the participants completed the Health Actions Diary devised by the researcher for a 2-week period (a copy of the Diary is provided in Appendix 1). The Diary consisted of two sections. The first section obtained information concerning the participant's age and sex, whether the person had any current diagnosed illnesses or disabilities, when the person had last visited a doctor and when or if the person had last been admitted to a hospital. The first section was completed on Day 1 of the data collection during an interview with the researcher. The second section contained questions concerning whether the person had experienced any illness symptoms on that day, whether the person had taken any actions and, if so, what the person had done. These questions were answered on separate daily sheets over the 14-day period.

It is important that the reader has a clear idea of exactly what was done. In the case of questionnaires, it is not usual to include the full text of the questionnaire in the main body of the thesis in the methods section. Normally, the questionnaire is included as an appendix. However, as discussed in Chapter 9, when presenting frequencies tables of responses to questions from a questionnaire, it is helpful to include the exact wording of the question, in some instances, as part of the results table.

In a qualitative research project involving interviews, it is highly appropriate to describe the interview schedule in the case of a structure interview or focus group and/or the themes covered in an unstructured interview. An example follows:

Each of the focus groups was presented with the same set of discussion questions by the researcher. These included:

- What would you say is the main thing you feel about being HIV positive?
- How have your friends reacted to your HIV-positive status?
- How has your family reacted to your HIV-positive status?
- How do you explain that you have survived your illness for the time that you have?
- Why do you think other people have not survived as long?

These questions were derived from an analysis of previously published discourses in the area of cancer research published by Smith & Jones H (1992, 1993, 1994) and modified for the present study by substituting HIV for the word cancer. As previously discussed, it is proposed to compare the discourses generated in the present study of people with HIV-positive status with those discourses generated by people with life-threatening cancers.

Of course, the above are abbreviated examples of what might be offered, but they give a flavour of what might make examiners smile. The examiner should be in no doubt about how the information was collected, what information was collected and why this method was chosen.

PROTOCOLS AND PROCEDURES

In this section, the researcher describes exactly how the research was conducted. In a higher degree thesis, this section could run to a couple of pages. Once again, in an Honours thesis, space dictates that it should be more economical of space. It is usual to commence with a brief description of your ethics approval procedures (see Chapter 8) followed by the nuts and bolts of the participant recruitment procedure. How were people contacted? How did you know where to find them? How was access obtained?

Ethical clearance to conduct the research was sought and obtained from both the Nuffield Regional Hospital Board and the University of Sussex.

The patients who attended the Rheumatology Institute during the month of February, 1999, were approached by the Institute's reception staff when they presented for their appointment at the Institute's clinic reception. The patients were handed a letter from the researcher that contained an invitation to participate in the research. The patients who wished to participate then telephoned the researcher at the University to indicate their interest in participation in the research programme. The researcher then arranged to meet at a mutually convenient time with the research participants. At this meeting, following signature of the informed consent form, the participant was then interviewed using the interview schedule described in the earlier section of this chapter.

While it is a commendable wish to spare the reader the gruesome details, it is important that the work is described to the level that it would be reproducible by someone else. Unlike in a journal article, there is plenty of space available in a thesis. Do not stint on the detail of how the study was conducted. The examiners will expect a full account of how the research was conducted.

THE METHODOLOGICAL DEFENCE

This section contains a detailed defence of the methodological approaches employed by the student in his or her research. It is a vital component of the fact and appearance of a high-quality research programme and thesis. This has proven to be a difficult section of this book to write because it cannot presume to predict the fine detail of the methodology of every thesis. Nevertheless, there are routine issues associated with various types of methodological approaches and problems.

The first area that needs consideration in the defence revolves around the generalisability of the results obtained by the procedures, tools and participants involved in the research.

Defence of sample size

Out of all the people who could have participated in the research, the researcher has generally selected a small number. This number has to be justified. One justification is the logistic defence. This runs along the lines of 'I would have liked to have more, but, hey, we all have to sleep at some point'. In academicese this could translate into some phrases like the following:

The recruitment of participants into the present research proved to be difficult as is often the case with clinical populations. To increase the sample size was not possible within the resources available.

This is marginally better than no defence at all. A much better defence in a quantitative study is a statistical one, based on the statistical power of the analysis and the required sample size. If you are reporting an intervention study, or one in which group means are compared, for example, involving analysis of variance, then in a higher degree thesis some attention to power is required. In an Honours thesis, a short reference to power issues is probably enough. If you do not know what statistical power is, then you need to read the following section and some associated references because it is very important that you understand what it is about. If you are performing a qualitative study, then skip this section.

Statistical power

In a study where there are tests of group mean differences (this includes most intervention and experimental studies), it is essential that the issue of statistical power is canvassed in the write-up. Readers will recall from their basic statistical training that when a researcher applies a statistical test, in addition to correct rejection of the null hypothesis and correct acceptance of the null hypothesis, there are two types of errors that can be made. These are the incorrect acceptance of the null hypothesis (a Type II error or miss) and an incorrect rejection of the null hypothesis (Type I error or false alarm).

The power in a study is the probability of (correctly) rejecting the null hypothesis when the alternative hypothesis is correct. It is defined as $1 - p$(Type II error). Cohen has argued that an acceptable value for power is 0.80 in any study. That is, when the null hypothesis should be rejected (there is a real effect) it *is* rejected on 80% of occasions. Or on the other hand, on 20% of occasions when there is a real effect, it is missed.

The concept of power is quite different from the α level (usually set at 0.05) in which the researcher can adjust the acceptable rate of false alarms, i.e. incorrect rejection of the null hypothesis (0.05 represents a 5% rate of false alarms, 0.01 represents a 1% rate). The reader will recall that reducing the false alarms, i.e. making the α level more rigorous by adjusting it, for example from 0.05 to 0.01, simply means that more Type II errors (misses) will be made. Many researchers are misguidedly obsessed with the α levels and forget about power. But not all the examiners, mes amis! Many grant applications now require a discussion of statistical power to be included in the application.

Cohen (1969) has devised a somewhat difficult to understand book of tables in which the desired sample size to detect large, medium and small intervention effects can be determined.

As Keppel (1991) has noted, the power of a design is determined by three factors: the significance level (α) chosen by the researcher (almost always 0.05); the effect size (this is not controllable by the researcher); and the sample size. It is really only the sample size that is amenable to adjustment by the researcher. So if you chose an inappropriately low sample size and hence low-powered study, you may be punished by an examiner if you do not discuss this issue in your analyses and their interpretation, particularly if you have null results. Indeed, if you have null results, i.e. no differences or group effects detected, then not discussing the statistical power of the analysis is a risky business.

Defence of participant selection method

While the sample size defence is more a feature of the quantitative than the qualitative research project, the selection of study participants is important in both. Most health sciences studies employ incidental rather than random sampling procedures. It has already been noted that a key feature of the reporting of participants is the response rate, i.e. the proportion of people approached to participate in the research who actually did so. If it is very low, say 10%, then the findings will and ought to be interpreted very differently from when the response rate was, say, 80%.

The key issue in participant selection is the representativeness of the participants with respect to the population from which they were drawn. One way of demonstrating this is to collect information about the participants and then compare this information with known characteristics of the wider population. If, for example, you are studying athletes but your group is older than the general population of athletes, this might have important implications for the interpretation of your results. Recovery times from injury might be an important facet of your study. You need to demonstrate to the examiner that you have considered these issues.

Defence of the research design

In a qualitative study, the interpretive methods chosen and the theoretical stance of the researcher need to be defended. Incidentally, defence does not mean a personal attack on the proponents of the other methods! The reader needs to know the stance that you have chosen and why you have chosen it. I personally consider that the defence of qualitative epistemology and methodology is more taxing than in a quantitative context because there is far less agreement about what approaches should be taken. At least the quantitative researcher has a more stable base on which to build an argument. Let us examine some of the more common research designs and how they might be approached.

Experimental designs

An experiment is a study where a sample of participants is randomly assigned to groups and then the groups receive different treatments. The goal of the experiment is to attribute the differences in the groups following the interventions, to the interventions themselves. If this can be done, then the experiment is considered to be internally valid (Polgar & Thomas, 1995).

There are many reasons why an experiment may not achieve internal validity. As outlined in Polgar & Thomas, Cook & Campbell (1979) defined a number of such threats including:

1. *History*. This refers to unplanned events that occur at the same time as the intervention. For example, in an exercise study, some of the participants may become ill with influenza, thus affecting their results.
2. *Maturation*. This refers to the phenomenon of natural changes in the participants over time. In a study of injured people, the injuries may spontaneously lessen owing to natural recuperation.

3. *Testing.* This refers to the phenomenon where the test procedure might alter the participants. For example, a series of exercise tests may have their own fitness benefit quite apart from the interventions.
4. *Instrumentation.* The measurement tools or apparatus may change during the course of the study, giving misleading results.
5. *Regression to the mean.* In this phenomenon, people who are chosen for selection into the study on the basis of extreme scores might 'spontaneously' improve or decline because of a measurement artefact.
6. *Selection or assignment errors.* In this phenomenon the groups, owing to faulty assignment to groups, may be different at the outset, thus giving rise to the artefactual appearance of post-intervention differences.
7. *Mortality.* If you have a large drop-out rate in your study, this may introduce group inequivalence similar to assignment errors.

Experiments can also be prone to various expectancy and social facilitation effects including the Rosenthal and Hawthorne effects if human observation is involved. The Rosenthal effect refers to the phenomenon where researchers may inadvertently alter their results to comply with their expectations. The Hawthorne effect refers to the phenomenon where research participants may alter their behaviour as a result of the knowledge that they are being observed. This is why blinding (the participants do not know the research hypotheses) and double-blinding (neither the participants nor the person administering the protocol know the research hypotheses applying to that particular participant) are employed in some experimental research projects.

Many of these threats to internal validity in experiments can be assessed through the use of a pre-test/post-test design where the groups are assessed before and after the interventions(s). If these threats could apply to your experimental design then you should specifically mention them in your methodological defence as well as in the results and discussion and the conclusions (in its limitations and strengths of the present study section).

It should be noted that a design involving the comparison of groups need not be an experimental design. For example, studies investigating health differences in smokers and non-smokers, where group membership has not been determined by the researcher, are not experimental by definition. Such designs are natural comparison or quasi-experimental designs. The basic weakness of such designs is group inequivalence on variables other than the grouping variable chosen by the researcher. This can be addressed to a certain extent by the intelligent application of multivariate statistical techniques.

Survey research

A survey involves the collection of data about the characteristics of a single group of people. This is often followed by an exploration of the associations between variables within the study. Such associations are sensitive to the representativeness of the selected sample. That is, if the sample is chosen in a biased fashion, the patterns of associations within that sample detected by the researcher may be at considerable variance with those to be found in a representative sample.

It is possible to employ a survey design to compare the characteristics of the participants with known characteristics of populations. This is one of the advantages of using standardised tests. A conventional approach to testing whether, for example, carers of older people were less anxious than people with the same characteristics who were not carers, would be to take two small groups, administer the test and compare them on the anxiety measure. This is actually a weak design because, with the small sample sizes, the power will be low. An alternative approach would be to put all the data collection resources into one basket (the carer basket) and to use standardised measures for which population (or very large sample) characteristics are known. Some advice I gave to one of my students on this matter concerning how to write up this issue appears below.

The present study involved the study of a single group of carers. It is useful to consider the methodological strengths and weaknesses of this design approach. One alternative way of conducting the study would have been to include some sort of matched comparison group (not involved in care-giving) in order to compare the responses of the two groups. This approach, however, has some flaws in comparison to the use of standardised items and tests as employed in the present study. In the instance where two small samples of participants are compared, high sampling variability issue is present in both samples. Thus it is difficult to reject the null hypothesis because of both the high within-group variability and also the high between-group variability caused by small n sampling conditions. The use of standardised tests and items from previously performed large-scale studies drastically reduces the sampling variation in one of the 'samples'. This permits a much more satisfactory test of the null hypothesis and between-group comparisons than the sometimes conventional small comparison group design.

In this particular study, the student used some items from the Australian National Health Survey conducted by the Australian Bureau of Statistics as well as standardised tests such as the Spielberger State Trait Anxiety Inventory, Profile of Mood States and General Health Questionnaire. This permitted the concentration of resources into the collection of one larger sample of participants who were carers rather than two smaller samples.

Defence of data collection methods

There is a rich variety of data collection methods available to the health sciences researcher including direct physical measurement, clinical observation, the use of self-report questionnaires and inventories, interviews including focus groups, and secondary data collection from documents and databases.

Direct physical measurements

The calibration of the tools used in the measurements needs to be carefully performed and described. Most physical measurement tools have published data concerning their reliability and validity. This must be included in the methodology and discussed in the defence. Below appears some discussion of issues that could be included in the defence of some of the major data collection methods employed in health sciences research.

Clinical observation

If the observation is performed solely by the researcher who also knows the research hypotheses and aims, then the methodologist's warning bells would be ringing loudly. There should be some attempt to study the reliability and validity of the observations, probably by performing a basic test–retest and inter-rater reliability study involving at least one other clinician.

In this study, the things to be observed and rated would be observed and independently rated by at least two observers and, if practicable, the same cases should be rated twice to test reliability. Otherwise the examiner may say that you are studying yourself and your outcome expectancies rather than real phenomena.

Self-report measures and questionnaires

One of the major problems associated with survey designs is the extensive use of 'home-grown' questionnaires with unknown properties. If there is an existing published inventory that deals with the same subject matter as the research questions with which the research project is concerned, then it is better to employ these inventories wherever possible (provided, of course, that it has satisfactory properties).

It should also be remembered that in self-report inventories people can lie ferociously about themselves. How do you know that they are not lying? Of course, in many research areas, it is polite not to mention this obvious fact. You cannot rely on your examiner being polite. In writing up results from self-report measures, it is useful to be careful in your use of language. For example, 'the participants claimed to have' or 'reported that', not merely 'had'.

Interviews

An interview is a conversation between the researcher and the research participant. The same issues concerning self-reports apply to a lesser extent because the epistemological position adopted by most researchers using interview procedures is that there is no verifiable external reality against which the participant's 'answers' can or ought be compared. However, in any interview, there is the recurrent problem of researchers imposing their agenda and perhaps their views upon the participants. As discussed in Thomas et al (1992), focus group discussions are less easily contaminated by an overly directive researcher.

Secondary data collection from documents and databases

The main issue associated with this method of data collection is data quality. How can the researcher be certain that the information collected is valid? This needs to be addressed in the defence.

Finally, when writing the defence it is important not to adopt an overly apologetic tone in its presentation. The point of the exercise is to demonstrate that you are aware that your research has limitations and that you have performed a thorough scholarly job of evaluating these limitations. It is not an exercise in saying, 'Please, please, I know that my research is worthless, but have mercy on a fellow health scientist'. Every piece of work could be improved. Maintain your balance in the critique of your own work.

8

Ethics procedures

In recent years, universities have become preoccupied with ensuring that all of the research conducted by their staff and students adhere to defined ethical principles and procedures. Some of this interest is altruistic and quality oriented. Other aspects of it include coverage for the university in terms of professional indemnity should someone be harmed as a result of his or her participation in the research. Parenthetically speaking, students should ensure that they are covered by the university's indemnity insurance and/or their own insurance in the case of a research mishap, as a personal civil suit from an injured party could be disastrous.

It is no-one's intention, but especially in the health sciences, for research participants to be harmed as a result of their participation. However, accidents can occur and unforeseen circumstances can arise. It should also be remembered that injury need not only be physical. Psychological harm or distress are every bit as real as a physical injury to the person experiencing them. Thus, the purpose of the ethics procedures is to minimise harm to research participants and to maintain their dignity and worth.

Most universities require the student to have ethics clearance from the University Human Experimentation Committee before any research work can commence. Do not be fooled by the name attached to the committee. Ethics approval is normally required before any type of data collection involving humans can occur, not just in experimental or clinical intervention research. Research involving interviews and survey questionnaires also has to be ethically vetted before it can be used. Only students using document-only research (provided they are not medical or confidential records) can avoid the requirement for ethics clearance.

If the work involves outside agencies, then you will have to obtain ethics clearance from each of the agencies involved as well. Strategically, it is useful to have the university's Human

Experimentation/Ethics Committee approval first to attach to your application for approval from the agency. Students who are negotiating their way through multiple Ethics Committees soon understand why so few multicentre studies are performed. Obtaining ethics clearance can be an arduous and monumentally time-consuming venture. It is not unheard of to have a 6-month turnaround from initial application to final clearance. If you can minimise your exposure to multiple ethics committees, it is advantageous to do so. Apart from the time aspect, it is quite common for different ethics committees to take exception to different parts of your protocol or to take different views about the same part of your protocol.

ETHICAL PRINCIPLES

Different countries and institutions have different criteria by which they evaluate applications for ethical approval. For example, in Australia, the National Health and Medical Research Council has a set of human experimentation guidelines and notes that describe the principles that have to be observed by researchers funded by that body. Many other institutions have adopted these guidelines. In the UK, the Medical Research Council has published guidelines that have also formed the basis for many institutional procedures. The situation in the USA is less uniform but the major grant bodies certainly have stringent ethical procedures and guidelines.

It should be noted that some ethics committees not only perform an ethical evaluation of the project but also examine the soundness of the research project itself. This is to determine whether the research is worthwhile and well designed. If they determine that it is not, then they may refuse ethics clearance on the grounds that to perform poorly designed research is unethical. Having such evaluations of your proposals can create dyspepsia from time to time, especially if the critique is not well founded.

Of course, access to institutions can be denied on grounds other than ethical grounds. If the research consumes clinical resources that are stretched or is likely to result in findings that may culminate in a black eye for the organisation, then do not be surprised when the answer is no. Over a period of 18 months one of my students tried at several hospitals to obtain clearance to videotape critical care nurses in action in order to analyse their decision behaviour. Presumably because of concerns about the possibility of filming clinician errors, access was denied on each occasion despite encouragement to redraft the protocol in ways that were suggested by the hospitals to meet their objections. There was never any question of filming patients in the protocol. This was specifically excluded in all versions of the protocol. In the end, access was permitted using observational methods and audio recording; no videorecording was allowed. Be prepared for protocol modification when using external agencies in your research.

COMMON QUESTIONS ENCOUNTERED IN ETHICAL CLEARANCE PROCEDURES

To determine the exact requirements of your specific institution or another institution from whom you need clearance, you need to obtain the specific forms. However, it is likely that you will be asked some of the following questions.

1. Is deception to be used?
2. Does the data collection process involve access to confidential patient data without the prior consent of participants?
3. Will subjects have pictures taken of them, e.g. photographs, videos?
4. Will participants come into contact with any equipment that uses an electrical supply in any form? e.g. audiometer, electrical stimulation, etc.
5. If interviews are to be conducted will they be tape-recorded?
6. Will participants be asked to commit any acts that might diminish their self-esteem or cause them to experience embarrassment or regret?
7. Will any treatment be used with potentially unpleasant or harmful side effects?
8. Does the research involve any stimuli, tasks, investigations or procedures that may be experienced by subjects as stressful, noxious, aversive or unpleasant during or after the research procedures?
9. Will the research involve the use of no-treatment or placebo control conditions?
10. Will any samples of body fluid or body tissue be required specifically for the research that would not be required in the case of ordinary treatment?

If the answer is 'yes' to any of these questions, then you will need to provide detailed information concerning the procedures and why they are necessary for the research.

You will be asked to provide full details of the research aims and hypotheses, the recruitment of the research participants and full details of all procedures to be employed during the study.

INFORMED CONSENT

A key feature of ethics procedures is the ability of the participants to deliver informed consent for their participation in the research. If you are dealing with people with cognitive impairment, or people who are not legally able to enter into contracts such as children, then their guardian or friend will have to give their permission. If you can avoid using such populations, I suggest that you do so. Obtaining consent under these conditions can be a logistical nightmare.

Each time a participant to the research is recruited, it is usually necessary to obtain written informed consent. The participant is presented with a statement of informed consent that describes the purpose of the research, discloses any potential harm to which he or she might be exposed as a result of participation and a reminder that consent can be withdrawn at any time. Complaints procedures are sometimes also described. The exact content of this statement needs to be determined with advice from the appropriate ethics committee for your study. The statement usually forms part of the application to the ethics committee.

For research involving an innocuous questionnaire or a non-threatening interview, these procedures can be over the top. Most ethics procedures are oriented towards high-risk clinical intervention research where there is a real risk of harm to the participant. For students who are performing low-risk research such as the completion of a questionnaire, I suggest that they include a statement like 'I understand that by returning the questionnaire, I have indicated my informed consent for participation in the study'. This may avoid the need for individually signed consent forms if your committee will agree to it. In any event, it is usually the case that anonymity is a requirement of the survey return. This clearly cannot be achieved with a signed form. The person is disclosing their identity by signing. Some universities have 'fast track' procedures for dealing with low-risk research.

ETHICS RECORDS

It is important that you fully document any 'incidents' associated with your research and that these incidents are brought to the attention of your supervisor as soon as they occur. Most ethics committees have reporting procedures for such events. It is also a requirement from most committees that you archive your data for a period of at least 5 years in case there are any queries at a later date. The harmful effects of some procedures may not become apparent for a substantial period of time, so it is important that proper records are maintained.

9

Writing the thesis results and discussion

The results and discussion constitute the major part of the original work that is presented in the thesis. These are very important components of the thesis. This chapter commences with a discussion of the design of the structure of the results and discussion chapters or sections within the research thesis. The organisation of the presentation of results and discussion within the thesis requires fundamental and important design decisions to be made prior to the commencement of writing. A method of organisation that overcomes some of the dilemmas as to where precisely certain discussions points should be made is presented within this chapter.

THE ORGANISATION OF THE PRESENTATION OF RESULTS AND DISCUSSION CHAPTERS

The location of results and discussion within the thesis often presents major difficulties to the research student. Have you ever had the experience where you have shown your work to someone, perhaps your supervisor, and then he or she has asked you about issues that you have discussed in other parts of the thesis? Perhaps you speculate that this reflects the likelihood of short-term memory loss resulting from excessive imbibing of the departmental port? Or perhaps it confirms your suspicions concerning the calibre of the person who has had the temerity not to 'get it' despite your efforts. Then again, it may be that the structure of the presentation did not meet the reader's needs. Maybe things were not located where the reader expected them to be and he or she could not find them.

A conventional results section or chapter involves the presentation of the results of the data collection without extensive commentary or integration with other findings or work. This involves a rather bare bones description of the outcomes of the study or studies. A conventional discussion section is much more evaluative and integrative. It attempts to weigh up the evidence supporting the answers to the research questions posed within the thesis.

There are essentially two main ways of organising the results sections or chapters in a thesis; either by data collection or by research question. The decision as to how to best organise this material is influenced by the number of studies that are to be reported in the thesis. If there is only one study, then matters are simplified. The presentation of the results section or chapter would then normally be followed by a discussion of the results. The discussion would normally be organised under the headings of the research questions where all material pertinent to the questions would be gathered together and discussed. Thus the core section or chapter structure of the thesis might look like this:

Introduction
    Background and overview of the research
    Rationale
    Literature review
    Research questions

Method
    Participants
    Tools and protocols

Outcomes of study
Discussion of thesis findings
    Research question 1
    Research question 2, etc.
Conclusions

However, as discussed in the thesis scope section in Chapter 4, theses often now involve multiple data collections or studies. This can create dilemmas as to how to organise the materials. Should each study chapter have its own discussion section? If this is the case, then how can the findings for the different studies be integrated?

It is conventional practice to present the research study results under the headings of the various data collections. Thus, for example, if you had conducted a survey it would be typical to report the results of that study as a whole in one location (normally a separate chapter) within the thesis. Thus the organising principle for this type of presentation is the activities performed by the research student. Each data collection activity or study is reported separately, perhaps in a separate chapter. However, while it makes sense to present discrete activities in this fashion, there is also the objective of directly answering the research questions that you have posed earlier on in your thesis. It might be that various of the data collections or evidence that you have assembled for the thesis impact on more than one of your research questions. Should not, therefore, the results of the thesis be organised under the respective research questions? But would this not lead to a fragmented presentation? These are fundamental document design issues that need to be resolved in any thesis prior to the commencement of major writing activity in these sections.

To resolve this dilemma, I recommend to my students that they organise their results by data collection or study in separate chapters or sections but that these are then discussed under the headings of the various research questions within a single thesis chapter or section. The final structure of the thesis is therefore affected by the relationship between the research questions and the data collection activities reported within the thesis. In some of the disciplines it was once considered that there should only ever be a one-to-one relationship between the research questions asked and the research studies performed, with no overlap. In a sense, if a study answered more than one research question or alternatively a question required more than one study, then this was seen as badly designed and executed research. In such disciplines the goal was to design small and elegant studies that perhaps manipulated one parameter experimentally and answered a small question uniquely in an elegant fashion.

However, the methodological and epistemological landscape within the health and medical sciences has changed substantially. With the advent of qualitative approaches and also the realisation that most interesting questions cannot be answered by a single study, this basic design approach has now changed somewhat. We now find that research projects may address the same research question by using several different methods and studies. This is sometimes called 'triangulation of method'. In this situation the researcher explicitly acknowledges that the method used to collect the research data may impact upon the research outcomes. Let us consider some examples of multistudy research projects and how they might be reported in a thesis.

I recently was involved in a study that was investigating barriers to the use of asthma management plans among parents of children with asthma. The researchers wanted to find out what the parents thought of the management plans and whether there were features of them that promoted low levels of adherence or militated against adherence. One component of the project involved a study in which focus group discussions were held with two groups of parents of children with recent episodes of asthma to discuss these matters. Several discussion questions centred on the research question. The focus groups were facilitated by myself. The discussions were transcribed and a thematic analysis of the barriers and facilitators to adherence to the plans as perceived by the parents was conducted.

This study was to be followed by a second quantitative survey in which a much larger sample of parents were surveyed using a structured questionnaire tool, the design of which had been informed by the focus group study. In the final write-up both studies were to be reported as chapters of the report, but the discussion chapter was organised using research questions such as 'What barriers to the implementation of the plans were identified by the parents?' as the headings under which the results were discussed. Thus the chapter structure minus all the other usual bits might look like as follows:

Introduction
Method and overview of research programme
Study 1: Outcomes of focus group study
Study 2: Outcomes of parent survey
Discussion of thesis findings
    Research question 1
    Research question 2, etc.

This structure allows for comparing and contrasting as well as integration of the respective findings from the different studies. It also clearly identifies the data gathering activities that took place within the research programme. It should be noted that the Study 1 and Study 2 results chapters included some discussion of the results, but did not attempt to integrate the results of each study with the other. This was left to the discussion chapter, in which the results were integrated with each other.

In another project, we were studying the impacts of problem gambling upon children and adolescents. Once again, a large-scale survey and small-scale focus group discussions were held with the research participants addressing the same research questions. In addition, an analysis of presentations at problem gambling services using a client record database of contacts was conducted. The three studies were reported separately within their own chapters but the discussion chapter was organised with the research questions having separate headings. The chapter or section structure might look like this:

Introduction
Method and overview of research programme
Study 1: Outcomes of analysis of problem gambling service attendance records
Study 2: Outcomes of survey of children study
Study 3: Outcomes of children focus groups
Discussion of thesis findings
   Research question 1
   Research question 2, etc.

Thus each study is separately reported but then the results are integrated in a combined discussion chapter.

In the context of triangulation of method, several different studies using different methodologies and different paradigms are designed and conducted in order to address the same research question. It may be that your thesis research programme does not utilise this approach and that your studies are quite independent in content. Whatever the outlook and epistemological position of the researcher, it is important that there is a clear relationship between the results of the study or studies conducted and the research questions outlined in the thesis. The reader also has to have a very clear picture of what data gathering activities took place within the thesis. The approach of presenting the basic results of each study in a stand-alone fashion but then combining the overall discussion into a single chapter organised under the headings of the research questions is a particularly effective method of designing the presentations of results and discussions in a multistudy context.

However, it is not the only method. There are circumstances in which the research questions may themselves become the chapter headings, if the discussion is particularly detailed and complex. For example, I recently had a student who had performed a large-scale interview study where she had covered several areas in an extended questionnaire administered to injured farm workers. She used the broad subject areas delineated by analysis of answers to the survey questions as chapter headings. In fact, she also initially had mixed her various data collections, a survey and analysis of clinical records, together within the same sections. It was my view that this structure confused the reader as it did not clearly relate to either the research questions or the data collections performed within the thesis programme. When the work was re-drafted it included a much clearer picture as to exactly what studies had been performed and their relationships to the research questions.

In order to ensure that the work performed within a thesis directly addresses the questions posed within it, I advocate the use of what I call a content method matrix. This is also discussed in Chapter 6. In this matrix the research questions are listed on the left and the studies or data collections that have been performed to address them are listed as columns on the table. An example of such a content method matrix appears in Chapter 5 (p. 44).

In constructing such a matrix, if you discover that some of your research questions have not been addressed then this is an important design flaw in your research programme. I do not suggest that you necessarily present this matrix as part of your thesis write-up, but it certainly is an important part of planning the presentation of the results in relation to the studies and data collections that you have performed. I have seen some quite effective method sections where a table (effectively a content method matrix) has been presented showing the relationship between the research questions and the data collection activities. This has worked very well.

Therefore the presentation of research results in a thesis generally involves the stand-alone presentation of the outcomes of each data collection in separate sections or chapters followed by an integrating discussion section or chapter in which the outcomes of the various studies are discussed jointly. It may be that the outcomes of your various studies and data collections give results that are consistent. This is good. However, it may also be the case that different components of your data collections give somewhat contradictory results. If this is the case then it is essential that the relationship between the outcomes of the various studies are discussed in detail. Therefore as a broad strategy I suggest the presentation of the results of the studies in a stand-alone form in separate chapters and then the presentation of discussion of the outcomes of the studies jointly in an integrated discussion chapter. I further suggest that a content method matrix is used in order to ensure that all available sources of evidence in relation to the research questions are presented and discussed. The matrix may appear as part of the overall method chapter or section.

Remember that the research questions posed in the introduction and the headings used in the discussion chapter and perhaps your conclusion should all be the same. Do not, for the sake of interesting variation, delete or add some research questions or rephrase them so as to not bore the reader. Boredom and adherence to convention is just fine. The whole point of a research thesis is to pose and then answer questions. They need to be the same ones! It is essential whatever design approach you take in designing the structure of the results and discussion that the structure is clear and navigable. Within it your research questions, the data collection(s) you have performed and their relationship must be crystal clear at first glance to the reader. Do not embed your study or studies and questions within thematic groupings that may be obscure to the examiner.

Enough of design, let us turn to the nitty gritty of presentation of the results and discussion text.

PRESENTATION DESIGN PRINCIPLES FOR THE RESULTS SECTION OF THESES

Successful theses share a number of design attributes. These include:

- well-presented tables and figures
- clarity of presentation of salient results
- reporting of qualitative studies
- good layout
- a logical development of the findings.

Let us discuss each of these in turn.

Well-presented tables and figures

Most theses, whether quantitative or qualitative or mixed in orientation, include tables and figures/graphs. These need to be well presented. But what does 'well-presented' mean?

The first feature of 'well-presented' is that if you have a specific style guide to which the thesis presentation is to adhere, then use it and stick to it like glue. The American Psychological Association Style Guide is used widely throughout the health sciences (American Psychological Association, 1994). It has hundreds of pages in which everything you may want to know (and more) about where to put your underlines and commas is outlined in grim detail. Some examiners really care about this stuff, so you need to show them that you care too. If you play your cards right, you can spend days of avoiding writing by doing this sort of thing.

Another feature of 'well-presented' is 'understandable on its own'. I think that every single graph and table in a thesis should have a title and axis labels that would enable it to be removed from the thesis, to be shown to an intelligent person on the street and understood by them. Far too many tables and graphs presented in theses are poorly labelled and obscurely presented to the extent that intelligent examiners wonder what on earth the message behind a particular graph or figure may be. Remember that most examiners will descend and ascend from your thesis document in a reasonably chaotic way, generally balancing this task with many others currently on their desks. What may seem logical and clear when the thesis is read linearly from beginning to end in one setting may not seem to be when the document is read in fits and starts. It needs to be dead obvious and clear, even when randomly accessed. Figures and tables draw the attention of the reader and hence must be the showpieces of your exposition and convey a message on their own.

Incidentally, if you are presenting frequency tables of responses to questions in a survey, I strongly advocate the inclusion of the question in its exact wording in the title for that table. For example, a suitable title might be:

Table 1   Frequency table of responses to the question 'Have you ever enrolled in a research degree?'

For the presentation of responses to multiple questions in one table, perhaps something like the format used in the following table example could be used:

A further feature of 'well-presented' is elegant simplicity. Do not try to include too much information in one table or figure to the extent that the clarity of the message it is intended to convey is compromised.

Table 2   Frequency table of problem gambling service client responses to the question 'Please indicate the impact the counselling has had for you in each of the following areas' (n = 200)

Problem area	Response		
	Got worse	No change	Positive change
Gambling activity	8%	3%	89%
Financial issues	4%	16%	82%
Family issues	5%	10%	84%
Relationship issues	12%	4%	84%
Employment	11%	26%	63%
Physical health	3%	11%	85%
Leisure use	4%	13%	83%
Legal issues	10%	0%	90%

Another way to present information simply is in a box, like the example box below.

Box 1 Demographic characteristics of Study 1 participants (n = 160)		
Sex	Male	36%
	Female	64%
Age (years)	Minimum	1
	Maximum	97
	Mean	47.2
	Standard deviation	46
Main language spoken at home	English	97%
	Not English	3%

The presentation of graphs is also an area that requires some design skill. I have seen graphs where there have been so many variables being presented that the bars for the variables were reduced to about 1 mm in width in order to fit them all in one page. I suggest that in graphical presentations that a maximum of two variables be presented in one graph. If in doubt, try the alternatives and market test them on some of your research buddies. If you need to provide an extended explanation of what they are looking at, you already have your answer about whether it needs changing. Simplify it! The figure on page 82 is an example of a simple figure that is easily understood.

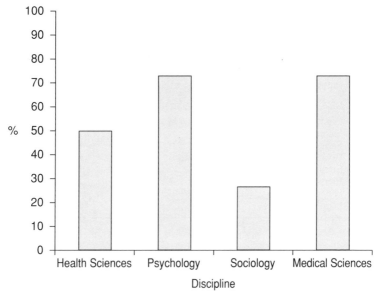

Figure 1   Percentage of PhD students enrolled at Mythical University in 1981 to 1986 who had completed within 10 years of their initial enrolment.

This leads me to the multi-page table. My best advice is to split it so that it fits on one page! Many thousands of theses and papers have been written without the need for multi-page tables. Yes, we understand that your data are unusually complex and difficult, but the challenge is to present them simply and elegantly to the reader. Multi-page tables are generally hard to follow.

Thus 'well-presented' in the context of figures and tables means 'adhering to the style guide', 'labelled so that it could be separated from the thesis and still understood' and 'simple and elegant'. Once again, I suggest that you look through the theses and journals in your area and imitate greatness.

Clarity of presentation of salient results

The results and discussion sections of many theses suffer from a lack of clarity. This is frequently a result of a lack of clarity in the mind of the author as to what he or she is attempting to convey. This is why I so strongly advocate the use of writing plans in all sections of the thesis, including the results and discussion sections.

The presentation of figures and graphs in results sections in theses follow a standard routine. Typically it goes like this.

The (exact title of your figure) is shown in Figure 1. These data show that…

The (exact title of your table) is shown in Table 1. These data show that…

Normally each 'result' would be followed by several sentences or paragraphs of explanation and discussion of the results. In a results section or chapter, the discussion of the results is typically somewhat minimalist and descriptive.

Reporting of qualitative studies

In the reporting of qualitative studies, there are far fewer standards available to guide the researcher as to how best to report and present the study outcomes. Frequently qualitative studies involve the use of interviews and the presentation of the 'results' involves intensive quotation from this material. Morse & Field (1995) provide a very useful discussion of the reporting of qualitative studies. They note that 'the most descriptive qualitative reporting appears to consist simply of quotations linked together with minimal textual commentary' (p. 173)'. Morse & Field are spot on in their description of bad qualitative reporting. Some thesis drafts consist almost exclusively of high-volume quotations from the participants with a bit of commentary. This will not work. The examiners will expect to see analysis. However, they will also expect to see evidence to support the analysis in the form of quotations from the participants.

In terms of presentation of qualitative materials involving quotations, I think the use of tables in which to present, for example, grouped exemplar transcript quotations can be a most effective method of presentation. In addition, programmes such as NUDIST or Ethnograph (these are packages that are quite frequently used to analyse transcript data) produce quite sophisticated outputs to show, for example, a category relation diagram to illustrate the relationships between coding categories as they appear within the natural speech and discourses of the participants in the research.

In the presentation of quotations or excerpts from the transcripts, there are some ethical issues that arise. The first of these is the extent to which transcripts should be edited to correct grammatical problems, lapses in expression and so on. Transcripts of natural discourses show how much meaning in speech is conveyed in the context in which the words are spoken. Divorced from this context, natural speech in the form of transcripts is chaotic. What we hear as grammatical beautifully parsed sentences in our heads are jumbled and often incoherent when in transcript form. Sentences commence from nowhere, cease without notice and have many grammatical mistakes. Should we fix the language? I think not. Consistent with the real ale movement, I think we should leave the 'flaws' in. As they say in sales pitches for leather goods, 'Certain of our products have marks. These are not faults. They are features of a natural product'.

However, identifying information should be edited out unless the speaker has specifically agreed to be identified. You need to be vigilant for this. We recently did a study of child protection clients and included the age and sex of the respondents alongside the quotations we included in the draft report. Because of the small numbers of participants, it would have been possible for these people to be identified, which would have violated the ethics protocols. Thus identification of the participant may be possible not only via their direct naming. In this case to adhere with ethics issues, deletion of text is justified.

Good layout

A high standard of presentation should be achieved with any document, but especially a thesis. If you are using a specific style guide, then these matters will be discussed in the guide and you should follow the advice contained within it. Many students fall into the trap of trying to make their thesis look like a desktop published report or magazine article, for example by using display formats such as multiple column text and so on. This approach will not necessarily be well regarded by examiners. Double spacing of text is usual for the reason that it permits the academic reader to put in comments without being squeezed for space. Also, it assists readability with what is often very technically complex and dense reading. In one or two cases, some of my students tried to obscure the fact that they had written theses that nudged the maximum word limit by manipulating the size of the typeface, for example from 12 point to 11 point, or squeezing the interline spacing. Grant bodies are now red hot on this sort of thing where applicants try to squeeze more words in by fiddling with font sizes and so on. My advice is not to do it. I myself wrote a very short PhD thesis of about 25 000–30 000 words and used triple spacing to try and hide it. Fortunately no-one seemed to notice.

A logical development of the findings

The order of presentation of the results and discussion should be carefully considered in the thesis design. It is important that the sequence of findings is logical and progressive. For example, in describing the outcomes of a study, it is usual to describe the participants first. In a qualitative study, there might be a detailed overview and discussion of the characteristics of the participants. As in a quantitative study, this might be provided in the form of some summary tables describing the characteristics of the participants. In quantitative studies this may involve group analyses, e.g. the participants were on average aged x years, y of them were women, and so on. In qualitative studies it might be more usual to provide a list of individual participants and describe their characteristics in an individual case-wise, rather than group-wise basis. For example, 'Doreen is a 45-year-old relinquishing mother who moved to the USA after 20 years in the former USSR'.

The best way to check the logicality of your sequence of presentation of results is to do a draft plan in which you outline the steps you are going to take in the presentation. This might look something like the following. Let us imagine that the study involved a survey of health service users to determine if there was an association between their satisfaction with various types of health services and their utilisation of these services.

First I will present some tables showing the demographic characteristics of the study sample including age, sex, cultural grouping and diagnostic grouping. Then I am going to discuss how this compares with the target study population using some data from the national Census for the social characteristics and then client records for the diagnostic grouping.

I will then discuss the issue of generalisability of the study sample using these analyses.

Then I am going to present the results associated with the first part of the questionnaire, which is concerned with people's current use of health services. I will group these under the headings:

- Use of hospital services
- Use of General Practitioner services
- Use of allied health services

I will present frequency tables for the various services grouped under these headings.

Then I am going to report the opinion data concerning the respondents' satisfaction with each of these services, using simple frequency tables, grouped under the following headings:

- Satisfaction with hospital services
- Satisfaction with Practitioner services
- Satisfaction with allied health services

Then I am going to provide some cross-tabulations of satisfaction with utilisation grouped under the following headings:

- The relationship between utilisation and satisfaction with hospital services
- The relationship between utilisation and satisfaction with Practitioner services
- The relationship between utilisation and satisfaction with allied health services

Then I am going to remind the reader of interpretational issues associated with correlations and the possible causal nexus. For example, does higher satisfaction lead to more or less utilisation or vice versa?

This is an example of how a results section plan might look. Remember that it is much easier to reorder and amend a plan than the real thing. The plan should be discussed with the supervisor and your other gurus and improved on the basis of their comments before you invest too much effort in writing. Which brings us to the discussion of the thesis conclusion.

10

The thesis conclusion

The concluding chapter of the thesis ought to perform a number of functions. It should review the outcomes of the literature review and how they articulated with the research questions; restate the major findings of the thesis and how they integrate with previous work; discuss the strengths and limitations of the research presented in the thesis; and propose future avenues of research and questions arising from the current work.

It has long been known in social psychology through the study of what has been termed the agenda effect or the serial position effect that the first and last components in any communication are the most influential for the judge or recipient. This principle also applies to theses. The concluding chapter, therefore, is a very important component of the whole thesis. It needs to be even more tightly written than the other components so that all the many threads in the thesis are woven into a golden cloth.

Let us examine each of the above mentioned functions of the concluding chapter and how they might be best addressed.

SUMMARY OF THE OUTCOMES OF THE LITERATURE REVIEW

In many theses, the literature review may be up to a third of the overall length of the thesis. It is surprising that many students do not even mention the literature review in their concluding chapter or section of their thesis. The literature review is supposed to be a comprehensive integration of current knowledge that identifies the knowledge gaps to be plugged by the research described in the thesis. That is, it should provide answers to the questions 'What do we know?' and 'What do we not know?' It should contain the arguments that lead into the statement of the research questions, i.e. the whole purpose of the research. If the literature review is not discussed in the concluding chapter, then one might ask, 'How can one discuss the answers without discussing the basis for the questions?'

A skeleton structure for this component might include statements such as the following:

In the present thesis, the xyz literature was reviewed. It was argued that certain studies in this literature had methodological problems that rendered their findings ... The abc literature was reviewed. It was found that ... On the basis of the overall literature review, it was concluded that ... Thus the status of ... was found to be unclear. The research questions addressed by this thesis were...

It is de rigueur to restate the aims of the thesis and the research questions in the conclusion. Do not worry about the readers being bored. If they wanted excitement they would be reading a thriller instead of your thesis. After 200 pages plus of academic meanderings, they need to be reminded of the plot! Tell them what it is. As previously discussed, it is folly to assume that the examiner will read the thesis in one sitting in a linear sequence. A series of random raids is more likely.

MAJOR FINDINGS OF THE THESIS AND HOW THEY INTEGRATE WITH PREVIOUS WORK

It is also not repetitious to provide a summary of the major components of the data collection and their outcomes. Although this is also done in the abstract and the particular results chapters, it is still a most worthwhile venture to describe the study(ies) and the outcomes. It is crucial that these outcomes are discussed with respect to previous work and findings. How was it similar to and/ or different from the findings of previous studies? The reader has to have a strong sense of where the new work reported in the thesis fits in with the old work, so that it forms a logical continuum.

In order to address the research questions, the following research was performed. In Study 1, 6 people with HIV were interviewed in a focus group. The purpose of Study 1 was to ... It was found that ... In Study 2, a quantitative sample survey was performed of 32 critical care nurses. The nurses were asked to complete a questionnaire including demographic items and the Attitudes to Physicians scale.

Statements such as the following need to be included in this section of the conclusions.

The research findings in the present thesis are at odds with those presented by Bloggs (1991), but are consistent with those presented by Nurk (1987). The present research demonstrated that...

The findings of Study 2 supported the predictions made by the application of the Health Belief model in that...

STRENGTHS AND LIMITATIONS OF THE RESEARCH

It is important that the student demonstrates a realistic appreciation of the strengths and limitations of the work he or she has done through communication of these issues in the thesis. Many theses simply present a statement about the limitations of the present work without discussion of its strengths. This is an unbalanced view of the work. If it was so poor, then why was it done in the first place? There are standard issues that require attention. These include:

1. *A discussion of the generalisability of the work.* This is affected by the selection of the participants and/or data sources for the study, the conditions and context under which the information was collected and the way in which it was collected. If the study employed volunteers as participants, what is known about the volunteer bias in the study. How might this have affected the results? Were there circumstances peculiar to the particular research that might impinge upon their application to other contexts and settings?
2. *The status of the methodologies employed in the research programme.* For example, if one used self-report questionnaires to collect the data then there are issues of validity, social desirability and so on that need discussion. If the researcher used non-standardised measures/instruments to collect the data then possible problems with validity need to be discussed.
3. *What was the research design?* What are the inherent strengths and weaknesses of such designs. How do these strengths and weaknesses manifest themselves in the present research?

FUTURE AVENUES OF RESEARCH

A glib 'further work is needed' is no longer an adequate conclusion to a thesis. 'Which work?' and 'How could it be done?' are questions that need to be answered in order to bring the thesis to a satisfactory conclusion. However, the thesis author needs to be careful that the questions proposed are not much more interesting and sensible than the ones he or she has studied! They should form a useful increment to the ones already answered by the thesis, not spear off at tangents or offer bright jewels and riches not provided by the present work.

THE PROCESS OF WRITING THE CONCLUDING CHAPTER

The conclusion must be the last chapter written in the thesis. This is because it requires all of the other information to be available for inclusion in it. I advocate a process of what I term 'deconstruction' to perform most of the actual writing process. By this, I mean taking apart the thesis elements and then assembling them into an abbreviated structure, a kind of reverse plan.

I believe that the first sentence of the conclusion chapter should be a brief statement of the goals and content of the thesis. Some examples might include:

This thesis reported the results of a study of carers of people with Alzheimer's disease. The purpose of the research was to discover whether the carers had elevated levels of psychological distress and use of health services when compared with people not involved in caring.

This thesis was concerned with the responses of people from non-English speaking backgrounds, specifically Greek and Chinese Australians, to primary health services. The purpose of the research was to discover whether ethnic background was a more important determinant of responses than demographic characteristics including the ages and sex of the research participants.

I consider that a reader who has not read any other part of the thesis should be able to grasp its basic content inside several sentences of the concluding chapter. Following on from the opening paragraph is the conclusion proper. As outlined above, I consider that the use of 'deconstruction' can assist greatly with the production of the conclusion.

The deconstruction process commences with the literature review. The task is to identify the salient features of what happened during the review and what was said. What was argued? Briefly what was the evidence to support your arguments? This information needs to be presented clearly and concisely. If you cannot identify clear and concise arguments from your literature review then this tells you something about the quality and structure of your review.

In terms of the length of this material, up to a couple of double-spaced pages (but certainly no more) should be adequate. There needs to be some substantive content in these pages, however. They need to be tightly written. Suggestions as to the possible content of this material are included in an earlier section of this chapter.

The second stage of the deconstruction commences with the statement of the research aims and an abbreviated description of the research performed to address them. This description should include details of the methodology employed. The reader who has not read the rest of the thesis should be able quickly to obtain the gist of what was done and why. It is imperative that the results obtained are discussed in relation to the previous research findings and that the status of the research aims is clearly and directly addressed. The quality of this integrating material, in my view, has a crucial impact upon how the examiners will receive the thesis.

Depending upon how you have structured the thesis, there might be a section that contains a methodological defence of the methodological choices you made in the execution of your research. Clearly these materials need to be elaborated and expanded in the section of the conclusions chapter that deals with issue of the strengths and limitations of the research presented in the thesis.

This is where the process of deconstruction ends. The final section of the conclusions of the thesis that proposes future avenues of research and questions arising from the current work is new material.

Students who have followed my deconstruction recommendations have produced near final draft conclusions sections in 2 working days. Most of the material in the conclusions should have been discussed in earlier parts of the thesis in various forms and hence the production of this material involves judicious editing in the main. If this material is not represented in earlier parts of the thesis, then this may present some difficulties for the reception of the work by the examiners because they will have difficulty in detecting the logical progression of the conclusions from the earlier material. Thus, the thesis will appear to be somewhat disjointed to the reader.

11

The thesis abstract

THE FUNCTION OF THE ABSTRACT

As with journal articles, the function of the abstract is to provide a summary of the basic content of the document that the reader is about to consider. However, a thesis abstract is a much lengthier venture than for a journal article, where the publishers often enforce quite strict word limits. It is not unusual for a thesis abstract to stretch to three or four double-spaced pages, whereas a journal article abstract might be one half to one page in length.

It is noted in the thesis conclusion chapter (Chapter 10) in this book that the first and last sections of the thesis are likely to have more impact and be more closely read by the examiners than other sections of the thesis. The abstract is literally the front door to your property and if it is in a shabby state of repair, then the expectations of the visitors are going to be adjusted downwards. Thus, if you are going to invest a special effort in the development of any section of the thesis, the abstract is a very good place to do so.

It is important that the abstract conveys succinctly and concisely: the area of interest, the knowledge gaps thrown up by the analysis of existing literature, the research aims and questions, the methodology to be employed to answer these questions and address the aims, the outcomes of the studies, their connection to previous results, the implications of the results and what future work might be pursued.

It is not good enough to provide vague and general statements such as 'The thesis concludes with a discussion of possible avenues for future work', or 'The data were statistically analysed' or 'Thematic coding was performed'. More detail is required. I advocate the following structure for an abstract following on from its functions.

HOW TO WRITE THE ABSTRACT

In the first sentence, the reader needs to know what the research was about. Some example lead-in sentences might include:

This thesis investigated the health problems of nurses working regular shiftwork in critical care settings.

or

The research reported in this thesis centred around the issues confronting gay men who had been HIV positive for periods of 10 years or greater but who had not progressed to AIDS.

This immediately orients the reader to the research issues under consideration. The second sentence could lead into the results of the literature analysis. Some examples might include:

Analysis of the research literature in nurse shiftwork revealed that the special problems confronting intensive care nurses had not been investigated in any systematic way. The few studies available were found to have significant methodological problems especially in terms of the biased samples employed. It was argued that this presented particular difficulties because of the pivotal roles held by such nurses in patient care.

Although many quantitative studies of such individuals have been performed, it was noted in the literature analysis that few studies had employed the tools of discourse analysis as outlined by Bloggs to examine the reactions of people in this situation. It was argued that the use of discourse analysis would provide important different perspectives of this important issue.

The reader needs to understand why the work is to be performed. In Chapter 5 of this text, some consideration is given to possible lines of argument for the support of a research programme, the identification of knowledge gaps being the most basic. These arguments should be included in a much abbreviated form in the abstract. Space is tight so a sentence only is required and available to do this. There should be an abbreviated statement of the research aims (and hypotheses if hypotheses are applicable to the research being reported).

The next port of call should be an abbreviated description of the research methods and protocols employed in the research programme. Examples of these might include:

At two large teaching hospitals with intensive care units, 40 nurses participated in a study of sleep disturbance and cognitive function over a period of 8 weeks. The nurses completed a daily diary in which they recorded any signs and symptoms of sleep disturbance. In addition at 2-week intervals, they were assessed using Silver's cognitive test battery.

Ten gay men who had been HIV positive for 10 years without any AIDS-defining illness participated in the research. The participants were interviewed each on four occasions using an in-depth interview procedure. At the first interview, a semi-structured interview schedule was employed. At the remaining interviews, an unstructured approach was adopted.

Having described the ways in which the study or studies were performed, the researcher should then describe succinctly what approaches were used to analyse the data and the outcomes of those analyses:

The data were subjected first to simple descriptive statistical analysis. These analyses revealed that 87% of the nurses had a sleep problem that would qualify as a clinical disorder according to the Sleep Society's diagnostic criteria. Correlational analyses revealed that nurses who had experienced a sleep problem in the 24 hours prior to the Silver's cognitive test had a score reduced to 50% on average of their normal score. This indicates that sleep problems may have a significant impact upon the performance of the intensive care nurse.

The interviews with the men were transcribed verbatim. These transcripts were then subjected to the thematic coding procedures described by Strauss and Corbin in their qualitative analysis text. This process was assisted by the use of the Ethnograph computer program. The major themes to emerge from the transcript analyses were: fear of death of partner, concerns as to the scheduling of retirement from the workforce … These analyses indicate that the long-term survivors who participated in the research have significant difficulty in adjusting to their longevity…

The next aspect of the abstract should include a statement concerning how the research integrated with previous work and also the research aims and hypotheses:

The results of the research program were consistent with previous work performed by Bloggs in which significant levels of sleep disturbance were found in general nurses involved in shiftwork. However, the present work is the first study to show these effects in critical care nurses. The hypothesis that episodes of sleep disturbance would be associated with impaired cognitive function was supported by the present research.

The themes identified in the participants' discourses in the present research were quite different from those studied in previous quantitative studies of men with the same characteristics. This implies that discourse analysis tapped quite different perspectives from those offered in the context of previous quantitative research.

The next step is to discuss the limitations and strengths of the research as ought to have occurred in the concluding chapter:

In the concluding chapter, it was noted that the study reported in the thesis had some shortcomings. The nurses recruited into the study were significantly younger and more inexperienced than the overall hospital populations from which they were drawn. This may have inflated the apparent effects of the sleep disturbance findings because the more experienced nurses may have had fewer symptoms. This was confirmed by the detection of age–impact associations within the participant cohort.

In the concluding chapter, it was noted that the study reported in the thesis had some shortcomings. There was some difficulty in locating men who had survived this length of time who were willing to spend their time in a time intensive research study. In fact 20 men commenced the study, but 5 withdrew before the first interview and 5 others did not complete the first interview.

The final section of the abstract should include a sentence or two about the future directions:

The thesis concludes with a discussion of future research avenues. It is suggested that a study should be conducted with more reliable measures of sleep disturbance with a larger sample in order to validate the findings of the present research.

The thesis concludes with the proposition that it would be most useful to conduct a comparative analysis of the discourses of people who have survived cancer on a long-term basis with those obtained in the present study in order to explore differences and communalities.

The above examples would need some integration and polish, but they provide some templates for the sort of thing that would normally appear in a thesis abstract. At all times the emphasis has to be on clarity and conciseness. The abstract needs to be all business.

12

The final production of the thesis

Once you have written the last word of the thesis and you have been given the go-ahead by your supervisor(s), you may think that the work is all over. On the contrary! You are about to embark on a fairly tedious full-time week or two of work physically to produce the thesis in a form suitable for submission for examination. In addition to the substantive academic text, there is a myriad of other components of the thesis that need to be produced. These are discussed below.

THE THESIS STRUCTURE
Thesis title page

Consult your university's thesis presentation guidelines for advice as to how to structure the title page for your specific situation. Normally, you have the centred thesis title with your name and any degrees you hold centred below it. At the bottom of the page you normally have a statement that reads: 'Being a thesis submitted in total (or partial) fulfilment of the requirements for the degree of Doctor of Philosophy (or e.g. Bachelor of Science with Honours) at the University of ...'. The month and year of submission of the thesis appear below this statement.

Table of contents

The table of contents should list all the major sections of the thesis document and all their page ranges. The skeleton of the table of contents can and should be produced in draft, but it can only be finalised with the actual page numbers when the rest of the thesis has been printed in final form. If you are an obsessional with five levels of headings in the thesis, I am sure you will want to replicate this in the table of contents. Just make sure that it does not exceed the length of the rest of the thesis. I suggest a maximum of two to three pages for this component of the thesis.

Declaration of authorship

The declaration is signed by the student and generally claims that the thesis is one's own work, all sources have been correctly attributed and that the thesis is presented in accordance with the university's guidelines and regulations for the degree.

List of publications arising from the thesis

If you have published from the thesis, then the examiners need to know about it! It may assist your progress through the examination. Aside from self-citation in the text of the thesis, the inclusion of a stand-alone list of publication(s) is an effective way of conveying this information. I advocate the inclusion of reduced photocopies of any published work as an appendix to the thesis. Include conference papers if you will, but I would not do this myself. Conference papers, unless they are refereed proceedings, have the same status as a public lecture, i.e. there is no particular quality control at most conferences and hence they are accorded a lower academic status.

List of figures and tables

The list of figures and tables shows the exact titles as they appear in the text of all the tables and figures included in the thesis. I cut and paste the titles from the actual tables and figures to ensure that they match exactly. You can include their page numbers to indicate their placement in the text if you wish, but it is a bit tedious.

Acknowledgements

The acknowledgements section has no substantive impact upon the reception of the thesis. But from an examiner's and supervisor's viewpoint it can be quite good for a laugh. Some students seem to draw upon an extraordinary range of (mostly) people whom they think should be thanked. Aunty Mavis, the cat, your spouse and even sometimes the supervisor receive some billing. It is polite to thank those who have substantively assisted you during your candidature. If you want to send special cheerios then this is best done in a separate document such as on a postcard or in a dedication page.

There is also a serious side to acknowledgements. This is when you have used other people's work and ideas. If you appropriate people's ideas in conversation and then write them in your thesis, the fact that you may have written them down does not make them your own. You have borrowed them from someone else. This is an area that requires considerable care. Acknowledgement of people's work that is already published is simple. You write this into the thesis. You can also incorporate direct acknowledgement of this material in the body of the thesis by citing them in the form of a personal communication ascribed to that person's authorship (e.g. Thomas, 1988, personal communication). If you do not use either of these methods to acknowledge the person's input, then a statement in the following form would be useful:

I am grateful to Dr Fred Nurk for his discussions and insights concerning the Health Belief Model. The section on this model in the thesis benefited (considerably) from his intellectual input.

However, in order to protect Dr Nurk from what may be on your part a total misinterpretation of the gist of his ideas, you need also to include a statement to cover all such acknowledgements:

Naturally, however, any errors in this document are entirely my own.

It is polite to seek the permission of people for whom you are going to include an acknowledgement, but it is not essential, especially if you include the disclaimer phrase above.

If you do not observe these niceties, it is unlikely that you will receive a writ and perhaps your God will not punish you. However, you may receive an academic backhander later when you do not need it. It is better to be safe than sorry as this type of activity can easily damage your reputation. You are not giving up anything by appropriate acknowledgement, but it is a very cheap and effective form of insurance against accusations of misconduct and impropriety.

Dedication

This is an optional page in which you can pledge your undying devotion to your goldfish. I think they are okay in books but a bit kitsch in theses. Nevertheless they make entertaining reading by others.

Abstract

This is really part of the substantive content of the thesis. How to write an abstract has already been discussed in detail in the abstract chapter of this book (Chapter 11). It should not exceed more than four pages of double-spaced text.

The body of the thesis

This includes the abstract, introduction, literature review, methodology, results, discussion and conclusions. The structure of the main thesis is discussed in detail in the respective chapters of this book. I do not propose to repeat this material here.

References

It is essential that every citation in the text of the thesis is matched with the correct reference in the reference list. The referencing standard should be chosen in conjunction with your supervisor. Many health sciences schools employ the American Psychological Association Style Guide as their standard (American Psychological Association, 1994). Most universities do not have specific standards for their higher degrees, reflecting the wide disciplinary differences in such matters. Most departments do have specific style requirements for Honours and Diploma students. As discussed in the style section of this book, failure to adhere consistently to the style standards in reference presentation is virtually a guarantee of (totally avoidable) adverse comment from examiners. If you use one of the electronic bibliographic packages, this should be an easy thing to do. Manual methods are error prone.

Appendices

The following items should be included as appendices to the thesis as a matter of course:

1. any survey questionnaire blanks or interview schedules not already in the main body of the thesis research
2. any publications arising from the thesis in photo-reduced form to save bulk
3. if you have quantitative data, an abbreviated listing of it. Some universities require all data to be lodged with the thesis. Others do not

4. if you have qualitative data, perhaps additional information
   concerning your coding structures or your transcripts,
   provided they do not resemble the size of the A–K section
   of the telephone book.

I advise against the incorporation into appendices of, for example:

- analyses that you did but did not include in the thesis;
- letters to people in the course of your studies;
- voluminous transcripts – say they are available upon request,
  if required;
- voluminous computer print outs – say they are available upon
  request, if required.

There should be a limited number of appendices, perhaps up to
four. If you have more, examine your inclusion criteria carefully.
This is not an art folder of your paintings at preparatory school.
If the material is important, then it should be in the main body of
the text. The appendices are the place to store materials that are
too voluminous for the text but that the examiners may want to
consult to clarify their understanding of the exact nature of the
protocols you used and the information you collected.

The exact order of the above extra-body components of the thesis
may vary from setting to setting. It is strongly recommended that
the thesis preparation guidelines and previous theses at the institution be consulted to determine the exact local requirements for
your thesis. If there are none, then I suggest consultation of one of
the relevant style manuals such as the American Psychological
Association Style Manual (American Psychological Association,
1994).

PREPARATION AND PRODUCTION OF FIGURES

Figures consist of flow charts, models, graphs, photographs and
other diagrams. Their design is discussed in the thesis results
chapter of this book (Chapter 9). In terms of the physical presentation of these items for the thesis, it used to be the case that they
had to be printed on bromide sheets instead of ordinary paper. This
requirement has now been dropped by most universities with the
advent of graphical computer packages and high-quality laser
printers. When dealing with photographs, it is probably better
physically to paste a copy of each photograph into each copy of the
thesis rather than use scanner technology and laser printing. To

produce high-quality images using scanning technology is a skilled venture and also a time-consuming one. Photographs are generally the only place where colour appears in the thesis. Coloured graphs are generally not presented in theses, often because the style standards, which are centred around cheap printing costs for journals, prohibit them. Because of the conservatism of some examiners, even when the style standards do not prohibit colour, I would not choose it. It is like turning up to a function in an Armani suit when everyone else is in their denim bathing costume. They may resent your stylishness and throw you into the pool.

DUPLICATION AND PRINTING OF THE THESIS

The submission of the thesis is generally a two-stage process. In the first stage, the student presents soft-bound copies for examination by the examiners. Once again, the exact requirements of the binding process vary from institution to institution. In terms of the numbers of copies required, you should add to the number required by the Graduate Studies Office one for yourself and one (each) for the supervisor(s), so that if any queries arise they and you are in a position to consult a copy of the version of the thesis that was actually submitted (somewhat to my amazement, I know of some students who have not provided a copy of their thesis to their supervisors). This generally results in a requirement of at least six copies. This means that the thesis has to be duplicated. Although it is more costly, I suggest the use of professional copying services to produce your copies. It is possible to photocopy your own copies to save money, but they do not look as professional as those produced by experts. It is also possible to print six original copies using a large-volume printer, if you have the word processing facilities necessary, but this is generally very time-consuming and very costly. For a large thesis, even with high-powered laser printing facilities, you are looking at a half day of actual printing time per copy. This is much slower than a photocopier and the per copy cost is generally two to three times that of the photocopier. Also, it can lead to errors.

PROOFREADING

Before you duplicate and bind anything, the thesis needs to be very thoroughly checked. It is useful to pause and note that the thesis has taken at least a full year, and perhaps many full years, to produce. It is foolish to compromise the reception of it by compromising its quality through rushing the final physical preparation. From the time you finish the actual writing and it is approved, remember to budget, including printing and binding time, two full-time weeks of your own time. If you do it in less time then you are exceptionally fast or you have cut some corners.

If you want others to be involved in proofreading, especially the supervisor, then you need to warn them in advance of when this is likely to occur and to budget for a reasonable period of time for them to do it. Reading a thesis, even for proofreading, is a major venture. It takes time and you will not win any friends if you take many months to produce the goods and then want a 1-day turnaround. It is sometimes useful to have an intelligent lay-person, perhaps a partner or spouse, to perform proofreading of the thesis. It is also possible to hire freelance editors to look over your work. You need to be careful about the extent of input from people other than your supervisor, for whom it is understood that there will be major input. The authorship declaration needs to be an accurate reflection of the true authorship of the material. Extensive input from a third party raises doubts about the authenticity of that declaration.

THE FINAL HARD-BOUND COPIES

As described in the following examination chapter, it is usual to have to perform some corrections on the thesis. When these have been made and approved, the thesis is then reprinted and hard bound. It then looks like your own (not so little) book. You can exercise your individuality in choosing dull maroon, dark blue or subdued green as its cover colour. It is polite to provide your supervisor(s) with their own hard-bound copies. They have invested many hours with you.

13

The examination of the thesis

THE SUBMISSION AND EXAMINATION PROCESS

The examination of the thesis is the culmination of a great deal of work on the part of the student and his or her supervisor. It can be literally a make or break exercise, so it needs to be approached with much preparation and care.

While universities and colleges vary in the exact details of the process, the general approach is pretty much universal. Honours theses are handled within the department in which the student is enrolled. Prior to the submission of a higher degree thesis, the student usually submits to the University Research and Higher Degrees Office a notice of intention to submit form along with a thesis summary designed to seduce the examiners into examining the thesis. The supervisor, often in consultation with other staff, is then asked to nominate a panel of examiners (perhaps two or three). A spare is also nominated in case one of the examiners decides to refuse the invitation to examine.

I consider it good manners and good sense on the part of the supervisor to approach the potential examiners before their nomination in order to determine whether they have the time and inclination to perform the examination. However, since their nomination has to be approved by others, it is, of necessity, a provisional invitation. Universities in general like to think that the student is unaware of the identity of the potential examiners. This is presumably so that approaches cannot be made by the student to the examiners in order to influence the examination. In fact, often the student is aware of the identity of some of the examiners for a variety of reasons. First, in most fields, there is a small number of potential examiners available and they may independently communicate with the student prior to examination. Second, the student at the end of the candidature ought to be approaching or exceeding the expertise of the supervisor in the specific field of the thesis and therefore, it is sensible for the supervisor to consult the student as to who might be a suitable examiner. During the process of the examination, it is a very bad idea for contact between the student and the examiner to occur. On some occasions, well-meaning but foolish examiners may approach the student about matters associated with the examination. If this occurs, the approach must be politely resisted and immediately reported to the supervisor. It is completely inappropriate for such contact to be made.

TYPICAL FORMAT OF A THESIS EXAMINATION

Most universities and colleges have a short one-page 'tick a box' form that is completed by the examiner to summaries his or her overall opinion of the thesis. This is accompanied by a short (generally one to three pages) qualitative unstructured report written by the examiner to support his or her opinion. The exact choices as to examination outcome that are available to the examiners vary from institution to institution, but most correspond to the following.

1. Passed with no further examination, perhaps with correction of a small number of typographical errors.
2. Passed with no further examination but some substantive changes that need to be made to the satisfaction of either the supervisor or the Chair of the relevant Examinations Committee.
3. Deferred, to be resubmitted for examination following changes of a relatively substantial nature.
4. Failed.

In the higher degree systems descended from the British model, procedures vary but it is common to have a face-to-face interview or viva voce examination associated with the examination. In systems descended from the USA, a thesis defence meeting is routine. In the Australian system, the entire examination can be a paper one with no dialogue at all between student and examiners.

If you are having a viva or thesis defence, it is vital that you are appropriately prepared. Almost certainly you will be asked to provide an overview of your work, the rationale for it, the literature you reviewed, details of the studies you designed, the rationale for the methods you chose, an outline of your results and their limitations. This is an activity that you need to practise.

Most departments provide venues for students to obtain practice in this sort of presentation such as in student conferences or the departmental colloquium. Take advantage of it.

EXAMINATION REPORTS

Examiners vary widely in the ways in which they structure their written examination reports. Some focus on the minutiae of typographical and formatting errors rather than on the quality of the ideas and arguments presented. (Which is why it is an excellent idea to give the nit-pickers very little to comment about by preparing the thesis so that it is as error-free as possible.) I have seen some outrageous things written in examiners' reports. Some examiners seem to delight in causing the maximum offence to their examinees. This is why the selection of the examiners is so important in the first place. However, this process is outside the control of the student. And, even when examiners are carefully selected, they can still do some unexpected and perhaps unfair things.

SOME OBSERVATIONS ON THE SELECTION OF THESIS EXAMINERS

In academic life, we all have colleagues who are irritable. It is my view that sometimes irritability and negativity can be confused with high academic standards. As a methodologist who has sat on higher degree committees for a decade or two, I have seen some woeful examinations where the examiner has made technical errors of major order. I remember vividly one student being victimised because he had deleted some discrepant points from his data that he attributed to instrumentation failure. One examiner seized upon this issue and attempted to portray the student as having 'cooked' his data. A review of most basic data analysis texts would reveal the ludicrous nature of this claim.

I also remember another examination where one of the examiners argued that the data should be treated as being at a lower level of measurement than the student had performed in his or her thesis. This is despite several dozen published articles, referred to by the student in defence of this procedure, in which the same procedures had been followed. The examiner was attempting to force this change against prevailing mainstream practice in the published international literature. Often being negative can be more an indication of robust stupidity than a sign of high academic standards.

In my view, if an academic colleague has a reputation for being difficult then he or she should not be selected to participate in the examination. The disruption that can be caused by unfairly intemperate criticism is not worth it. This is not to say that the examination should be 'cooked' by having only academic 'sweethearts' involved. The prize has to have some value. In terms of maximising future job prospects and international exposure, a fair and well-known examiner of international standing, provided the thesis is well received, can have a positive effect upon the student.

RECONCILIATION OF EXAMINERS' REPORTS

It is quite common for the university to receive different opinions from the examiners concerning the same thesis. Very often, the opinions are discrepant in a minor way. Sometimes, there is a major discrepancy. In most institutions, the relevant Graduate Studies Committee considers the examiners' reports and attempts to reconcile them. The supervisor may be asked to comment on the reports. In most British system institutions, the student is specifically excluded from this process.

If revisions are required, the Graduate Studies Committee, acting on the advice of the supervisor, will prepare a consolidated set of revision guidelines drawn from the examiners' recommendations. This avoids the problem of the student having to deal with the reconciliation of conflicting suggestions from the examiners. Also, the Graduate Studies Committee will sometimes reject the specific suggestions of one or more of the examiners. However, as the examiner has been nominated by the university as an acknowledged expert in the field, it is inconsistent to reject totally his or her opinion.

HOW TO DEAL WITH REVISIONS

The first step in the process is to put your annoyance to one side. Yes, you are probably smarter than Professor Bloggs, your examiner. Yes, he or she may not have fully grasped the subtlety of your argument. Yes, the suggested amendments may not be sensible in your opinion. However, all this forgets one thing. You are the student and you want the degree.

There is also the possibility that the examiners made valid criticisms no matter how inconvenient or improbable this seems. To get the degree, you have to do what they want. You may as well smile, or at least mildly grimace, while you are doing it. I suggest you count to 10 000 and if you are still angry, do it again until you are not. Then commence the amendments. Thesis revisions need a clear and not a sore head.

A second thing to avoid is recriminations with the supervisor. The supervisor is the coach. You are the player. If the referee rules that you dropped the ball, it is pointless to attack the coach. You will need the coach in a cooperative mood to assist with the thesis revisions.

Most examiners' reports and the associated revision guidelines are clear about what they require. If there are things that are not clear in the revision guidelines, then you should discuss them with your supervisor. Once again, remember your goal is to get the degree. If you think the revisions required are not sensible, then write a paper about the issues, *after* you have made the changes as specified, and send it off to a journal. I guarantee it will not be published. In 5 years' time, you will not care about any of it. You will have the degree, and that is what counts.

14

Publications and the thesis

The ultimate outcome of a research project should be the communication of the results to other members of the relevant research and clinical practice communities as well as the participant community. Methods of communication include the professional/ scientific conference, publication in the form of a journal article, book chapter, research monograph or even a book. An additional method of communication that is rarely considered is the popular press. Each of these methods of communication is to be discussed. However, before this discussion occurs, it is useful to discuss academic authorship issues and conventions.

ACADEMIC AUTHORSHIP CONVENTIONS

In the world of academia, there are many conventions and rules that apply to the recognition of academic contributions to intellectual work. Unfortunately for students and supervisors these conventions are not well documented and may vary from discipline to discipline. For example, in the medical sciences it is the rule to find large groups of people involved with the authorship of scientific papers. In the humanities, such goings on are sometimes viewed with almost suspicion, with the sole researcher very much more prevalent. I have heard some academics wax lyrical about how could it possibly be that six people have contributed to a paper. It is my experience that such individuals have never worked in large teams. Maybe this is because no-one ever invited them! Notwithstanding personal positions on this issue, the specific expectations and rules governing publications activity in these contexts can vary.

I remember a very amusing (and I swear true) story told by an academic social sciences colleague sitting on a national medical research council along with one of her medical colleagues. She glanced across and noticed that her colleague was going through one of the applications and putting a red pen through various of the publications of one of the principal investigators. She asked, 'What are you doing?' He replied, 'I am just going through and deleting all the sole authored publications!' 'Whatever for?', she asked. 'Well, the work must be hopeless, since no-one else has been prepared to put their name to it!' Most social scientists spend their careers trying to repel all boarders, so it was inconceivable to her that the medical scientist could have adopted this position. This is my first sole authored book, so I am a little worried about this anecdote. It neatly illustrates the differing expectations concerning authorship in different disciplines.

It is pertinent to forget about the student issue for a moment and consider the wider conventions that apply when academics work together. If one is working in a team context as an academic, it is rarely claimed that the work is uniquely one's own and this is reflected in the publications emanating from the team. In the teams in which I have worked, prior to the design of the research programme, I have generally instituted a discussion of who is going to write what papers and the first authorships are allocated at that point. I ensure that each person is represented at least once in that position.

Given that experienced academics interact and behave in this way, this has implications for student publications. The student, even with a solo supervisor, is part of a two-person team with the supervisor. If there are more supervisors, then the team is enlarged. In a non-student collaborative setting, it would be amazing if there were regular meetings between academic staff about a research programme over a period of years and this then did not translate into recognition of the academic input of each person by the way of inclusion on the authorship list of published work arising from the research programme. With a student, the level of input and advice from the supervisors usually exceeds many times over that which would be provided when working with other academic colleagues.

Thus, my basic argument is that work published from the thesis ought properly to include the names of the supervisors. However, my personal position is that the student must always go first. To my mind, the publication of materials collected by students without inclusion of the students as co-authors is completely unacceptable. I also try where it is possible to involve students in publication activity as junior authors outside the thesis topic as part of the academic apprenticeship.

However, I have also observed instances of what I would term questionable activities on the part of both students and academic staff. To meet on a weekly basis with a supervisor to have detailed discussions about the research programme and to then claim that the work you have presented is entirely your own by publishing it on your own is a preposterous position in my view. With academic colleagues this situation would not be tolerated for one moment, yet some students feel put upon if they are required to reflect the input of their supervisor(s) in the co-authorship of material to which they have all substantively contributed.

Publication is the coin of the academic realm. If you have a strong psychological need to have all the coins in your own pocket, then you should go into business not academia.

I accept that my views may be at odds with those of the reader and that this is a controversial matter. Whatever the situation, it is important that these issues are resolved early on or before the commencement of the candidature. As health scientists, I am sure we all agree that prevention is better than cure.

WHEN SHOULD PUBLICATION FROM THE THESIS OCCUR?

In the context of an Honours programme, it is virtually impossible to publish the work during the candidature. The time lines are too compressed. In the context of a Masters or PhD, programme, publication within the candidature is possible. There are several reasons to consider publication during candidature. These include:

1. *External validation of the work prior to examination.* Nothing concentrates an examiner's mind more than a raft of articles appearing at the back of the thesis. This is an indication of thesis quality from leaders in the field of work. It is a brave examiner who would give a much-published candidate a hard time at examination.
2. *Publicity and improvement of job prospects.* If the student intends to use his or her degree to improve future job prospects, whether in academia or outside it, the production of high-quality publication material acclaimed by peers is a useful venture.

3. *As a means of completing the writing of the thesis*. A thesis can be a very long document indeed. It is helpful to segment the writing task into manageable chunks. However, it should be recognised that journal articles, in particular, are generally a much abbreviated form of what is required and expected in a thesis. One could not normally just string together several articles to form a thesis. Additional material is required. However, to have the framework is certainly highly beneficial.

It also has to be noted that publication is not an automatic activity. Lots of work is never accepted for publication. Publication is a prize that is worth winning because it means something.

CONFERENCE PRESENTATIONS

Conferences can be very useful venues for students because they are highly interactive. Leaders in the field display their wares and they can be queried about their work. This is expected and invited. Presentation at a conference is a worthwhile venture.

Most conferences advertise a considerable period in advance for prospective presenters to send in an abstract or summary of the work they might like to present at the conference. The conference scientific programme committee then vets the abstracts according to their selection criteria and if they like yours, you will be invited to present. Some conferences have special sections for research students. Students are also often asked to present their research proposals to departmental seminars or colloquia. This is also a useful experience.

Preparing for the presentation

In order to prepare for the presentation, it is necessary to consider the characteristics of the audience in attendance, the format of the presentation including the method and length of the presentation.

The target audience is an important guide to the preparation of the presentation. If the audience is predominantly non-specialists in the topic, then some simple explanations of key concepts would be useful. If the audience are specialists then simplicity in the presentation may provoke negative reactions. The language and detail of explanation must be pitched at the audience.

At scientific meetings, most presentations involve speeches accompanied by visual material such as slides or overheads. Some conferences have separate poster and display sections, where presenters provide a poster prepared according to the meeting's specifications and are allocated a time or times at which they stand alongside it, to answer any questions and perhaps to give a short speech. The standards in poster presentations at some meetings are now very high with extensive use of colour text, photographs and graphics. A bit of white paper with coloured ball point pen will not do.

It is *vital* that your presentation fits within the allocated time. Most meetings have strict chairpersons who will cut you off at the prescribed time no matter whether you have finished or not. The format for meetings varies from meeting to meeting. Some have questions at the conclusion of each paper. Others have group papers and have a common question session at the end. Ensure that you fully understand the format of your meeting before you go to it.

Most verbal presentations consist of a speech and accompanying slides or overheads. Presenters vary in their preferences about whether they have a word-for-word prepared speech or a set of notes to which they speak. Many use their slides or overheads to prompt their speech. It is better not to read a document to the audience unless it is absolutely necessary. The classically bad presentation involves someone reading word-for-word a prepared speech in a dull monotone, never looking up to see the audience. Remember that the audience may contain some of your future examiners!

There are certain features of good presenters. People want to feel that the presenter is communicating with them. If the presenter does not ever look at them, how can one obtain a sense of engagement? So, look around at the audience! Good presenters adopt a relaxed posture and speak in an interesting and animated fashion. Show the audience that you care about your topic.

The preparation and presentation of slides and overheads

The expectations is that slides/overheads will be printed, preferably in colour. Most universities now have the technology to produce high-quality overheads and there are many commercial services that can also do this. At large conferences, the use of slides is now fairly standard, whereas at smaller meetings, overheads are more common.

There is a wide range available of computer-based presentation graphics products. The most commonly used one is Microsoft® Powerpoint®. A common error in presentation of slides and overheads is to have too many points on one slide. As a rough guide, three to five points in each slide should be sufficient. In terms of the number of slides, this, of course, depends upon the length of time allowed for the presentation. A common error is to attempt to have too many slides or overheads in the presentation. In lectures, I use 12 per hour, but conference presentations are more frenetic, so this number might be used in a 15-minute presentation. I have seen some colleagues present 60 slides in a 15-minute presentation. This went over badly because people could not keep up.

Slides and overheads should be readable from all parts of the room in which the presentation is being given. The best way to determine this is to have a trial run in a similar room and see if they are readable. The audience will become unsettled if they cannot read your material. I am sure you have attended the odd execrable lecture where the lecturer has lost the audience because of poor presentation.

Many lecture theatres now have facilities for the projection of slides from laptop computers. If you are going to use this approach, have a backup set of slides or overheads with you. Do not walk in front of your slides when presenting them.

Practising the presentation

Practice of the presentation is essential. Some performance anxiety is normal for presenters. No doubt you have your own ways of dealing best with anxiety. Remember that you know your own work best. People are at the meeting to have the benefit of your expertise, so try to keep your anxiety under control.

Suggested slide headings and contents in a conference presentation

The suggested headings and contents for slides in a standard conference or scientific meeting presentation is provided in the following Table below.

Slide(s) title(s)	Contents
Title	Title of research, name of presenter and affiliation, names of other investigators
Background/Introduction	Previous work in the area is described, knowledge gaps described, what we know and what we do not
Why do this work?	Rationale for this work presented
Research aims	List of aims/research questions
Methodology	Description of participants, research tools, schedules used, description of research protocols provided
Results	Presentation of research findings, under headings of questions if possible
Summary of findings	A list of the questions and their answers
Where next?	What should be done next to advance the work
Some cautions	A clear statement of strengths and weaknesses of the work

JOURNAL PUBLICATIONS

The most common method of dissemination of results is through journals. Academic journals come in a hierarchy of quality, ranging from the internationally acclaimed to less well-known local journals. This hierarchy generally corresponds to the ease with which authors can have their work accepted for publication in the journal. Some international journals have rejection rates of 80% and greater, which means the work has to be highly regarded by the whole panel of reviewers to be accepted. Good-quality journals are refereed. That is, when work is submitted for consideration for publication, it is then sent to several independent reviewers for assessment. Some of the lesser quality journals do not have an independent reviewer process, or if there is a review process, it may be quite perfunctory involving in-house reviewers and perhaps only one reviewer. It is difficult to evaluate journal quality objectively, but there have been some attempts to do so by various academic bodies who have attempted to quantify quality aspects of academic output as well as pure quantity.

Submission of work to a journal for publication is an exciting and risky business, especially with the high rejection rates associated with some journals. Also, there is the certainty that your work will be criticised. However, the higher degree student should not view negative reviewer comment as an attack on his or her self-esteem but rather as free assistance towards improving the work. Journal reviews, as with thesis examinations, are largely a matter of opinion. Submission to a journal is a useful way of obtaining independent opinions about possible strengths and weaknesses of the thesis, prior to its final examination. This is not to say that all the reviewers' comments should be taken as good advice. You should discuss any reviews with your supervisor.

The structure of journal articles

Individual journals have their own instructions concerning how to prepare articles for consideration for publication. These should be consulted prior to drafting.

Most journal publications follow a structure with associated functions similar to the one below:

Title

The title provides an abbreviated description of the article content. The title must accurately convey the contents of the article in very few words.

Abstract/summary

The abstract provides a short summary of the content of the article; this is also used in electronic abstract databases such as Medline. Abstracts may range from 100 to 300 words, depending upon the journal. The abstract should be particularly polished as it is very widely disseminated.

Introduction

The introduction provides an overview of the research context for the work including a literature review, rationale for the work presented and a clear statement of the research aims to be addressed by the article.

Method

The method provides a description of the research participants and how they were selected and the research protocols that were employed in the study.

Results

The results section provides a description of the findings of the research. Results generally have very little commentary within them in a journal article.

Discussion

The discussion section provides a discussion of the answers to the research questions.

Conclusion

The conclusion provides an analysis of the work's strengths and weaknesses, what it means and what should be done next.

BOOK CHAPTERS AND MONOGRAPHS
Contributed works

It is a great honour to be invited to write a chapter in a book and this is quite unusual for a research student. It is a recognition of expertise that is generally only awarded to academics with an international reputation in their field. A book chapter normally contains a large integrative state-of-the art review rather than the presentation of primary empirical work, although this can occur in some instances. Depending upon the requirements of the editor, book chapters are generally about double the size of a journal article. This permits more depth and breadth of coverage than would normally be possible in a journal article.

Monographs

Many academics set out to write the great academic masterpiece. Few complete the task. This is, in part, because a decent sized book has about two to three times the word count of a PhD. At this point, would you feel like writing your PhD and then doing another one for good measure? A book takes a lot of effort to write. Also, you need to have a broad and deep knowledge of the topic in which you are writing. In most research programmes, depth is achieved but breadth is not. Research theses generally make for execrable books. My suggestion to a student who feels that their thesis should be published in the form of a book, especially if they have not written a lot before, is to lie down until the moment passes.

PUBLICATION IN THE POPULAR PRESS

This form of publication is rarely used by academics. I believe that this reluctance is because of the possibility of being branded as populist by other academics and because academics believe that their work will not be of interest to people in the general community.

Most universities have public relations and information offices that can assist you with the preparation of material suitable for distribution to the popular press. Another method of making contact is to contact the journalist responsible for the health and sciences areas in the news outlet.

It is important that you do two things in your discussions with the journalists. First, insist that everyone involved in the research is acknowledged. Tell them that if this does not happen, then you stand to be in a lot of trouble. I have been involved in instances where one academic in a large research team has contacted the media and the subsequent report has read as if he or she had done all the work unaided. This creates unnecessary bad feeling. Second, make sure that the claims made by the journalist are not extravagant. Your reputation could be damaged if you are announced under a headline 'Miracle Cure for Cancer' when what you did was to conduct a focus group with people with cancer. Ask to see the release or article before it is published to check it for factual accuracy.

Thus, there are many possibilities for publication of work from the thesis. As outlined above, there are many positive benefits that flow from participation in the publication process, even if the work is not ultimately accepted for publication. If the work is accepted, then this has substantial positive benefits for the examination outcome.

15

The last word

I have always found it difficult to know what to say at the end of a book or thesis. I have a theory that the last sentence in a thesis accounts for more agony than any other sentence, closely followed by the first one. So I have decided to finish my little book with some suggestions for your last sentences in order to relieve your stress and anxiety.

For those of you who are biblically inclined perhaps a few references to Armageddon or the Apocalypse would do the trick. If you like the X-Files, perhaps 'the truth is out there' might be appropriate. You could always try the *Tale of Two Cities* 'tis a far …' or some such. If you are a bit scientific, you could try babbling on about Newton's pretty stones on the beach and how you wish you had not thrown them at your house windows. Maybe you could talk about how your ugly hypotheses were ruined by beautiful facts. Maybe you could even try 'Frankly my dear, I don't give a damn'. The possibilities are limitless.

Since it was so long ago that I wrote my own PhD thesis (and it is a memory that I try to suppress), I decided to see what I wrote. It reads:

The initial steps taken in the present thesis could be developed into a better typology for judgement tasks and types of judgement models.

This is woeful. No wonder I have not read it since I wrote it.

I hope that this little book will help you with your thesis completion.

References

American Psychological Association (1994) *Publication manual of the American Psychological Association*, 4th edn. Washington DC: American Psychological Association.

Booth A.L. & Satchell, S.E. (1996) British PhD completion rates: some evidence from the 1980s. *Higher Education Review* **28**, 48–56.

Cohen, J. (1969) *Statistical power analysis for the behavioral sciences*. New York: Academic Press.

Cook, T.D. & Cambell, D.T. (1979) *Quasi-experimentation: design and analysis issue for field setting*. Boston: Rand McNally College Publishing.

Department of Education, Training and Youth Affairs (1999) *New knowledge, new opportunities*. Canberra: Ausinfo.

Holmes, T.H & Rahe, R.H. (1967) The social readjustment rating scale. *Journal of Psychiatric Research* **11**, 213–218.

Keppel, G. (1991) *Design and analysis: a researcher's handbook*, 3rd edn. Englewood Cliffs, NJ: Prentice-Hall.

Minichiello, V., Aroni, R., Timewell, E. & Alexander, L. (1995) *In-depth interviewing*, 2nd edn. Melbourne: Longman.

Morse, J.M. & Field, P.A. (1995) *Qualitative reserach methods for health professionals*, 2nd edn. Sage: Thousand Oaks, CA.

Office of Scientific and Engineering Personnel (1990) *The path to the Ph.D.: measuring graduate attrition in the sciences and the humanities*. New York: National Academies Press.

Office of Scientific and Engineering Personnel (1997) *The path to the Ph.D.: measuring graduate attrition in the sciences and the humanities*. New York: National Academies Press.

Polgar, S. & Thomas, S. (1995) *Introduction to research in the health sciences*, 3rd edn. Melbourne: Churchill Livingstone.

Thomas, S.A., Steven, I., Browning, C.J., Dickens, E., Eckermann, L., Carey, L. & Pollard, S. (1992) Focus groups in health research: a methodological review. *Annual Review of Health Social Sciences* **2**, 7–20.

Annotated thesis writing and research bibliography

American Psychological Association (1994) *Publication manual of the American Psychological Association*, 4th edn. Washington DC: American Psychological Association.
A good book on how to look after the commas.

Bowling, A. (1991) *Measuring health: a review of quality of life measurement scales*. Philadelphia: Open University Press.
A useful guide to health measurement scales focusing on quality of life measures.

Bowling, A. (1995) *Measuring disease*. Philadelphia: Open University Press.
A useful guide to health measurement scales focussing on measures of disease.

Bowling, A. (1997) *Research methods in health: investigating health and health services*. Buckingham: Open University Press.
A useful introduction to research methods in health service evaluation.

Crombie, I. & Florey, C. (1998) *The pocket guide to grant applications*. London: BMJ Books.
A very good guide for writing grants and applications. Comes with software.

Cryer, P. (1996) *The research student's guide to success*. Buckingham: Open University Press.
An interesting view of student life in Britain. Worth a look.

Delamont, S., Atkinson, P. & Parry, O. (1997) *Supervising the PhD: a guide to success*. Bristol: SRHE and Open University Press.
A guide to the research thesis from the viewpoint of the supervisor. Some useful ideas.

Denzin, N.K. & Lincoln, Y.S. (1994) *Handbook of qualitative research*. Thousand Oaks, CA: Sage.

A comprehensive account of qualitative research. Very lengthy read.

DeVellis, R. (1991) *Scale development: theory and applications,* vol. 26. Thousand Oaks, CA: Sage.
A very useful little book on scale development.

Greenhalgh, T. (1997) *How to read a paper: the basics of evidence based medicine.* London: BMJ Publishing Group.
One of the very good BMJ series.

Hawe, P., Degeling, D. & Hall, J. (1995) *Evaluating health promotion: a health workers guide.* New South Wales: MacLennan & Petty Pty Ltd.
Widely cited and useful introduction.

Henry, G. (1990) *Practical sampling,* vol. 21. Thousand Oaks, CA: Sage Publications.
One of the Sage series. Very good for the qualitative researcher.

Jenkins, S., Price, C. & Straker, L. (1998) *The researching therapist.* New York: Churchill Livingstone.
A useful introductory text with some useful sections on research student activity, and presentations.

McDowell, I. & Newell, C. (1996) *Measuring health: a guide to rating scales and questionnaires,* 2nd edn. New York: Oxford University Press.
Another useful guide to standardised measures.

Minichello, V., Aroni, R., Timewell, E. & Alexander, L. (1996) *In-depth interviewing,* 2nd edn. Melbourne: Addison-Wesley Longman Australia.
A useful practical guide to interviewing.

Morse, J.M. & Field, P.A. (1995) *Qualitative research methods for health professionals,* 2nd edn. Thousand Oaks, CA: Sage.
A good, simple, and accessible, qualitative book.

Norton, P., Stewart, M., Tudiver, F., Bass, M. & Dunn, E. (1991) *Primary care research: traditional and innovative approaches,* vol. 1. Thousand Oaks, CA: Sage.
Discussion of epistemology of health/medical research.

Patton, M.Q. (1990) *Qualitative evaluation and research methods,* 2nd edn. Thousand Oaks, CA: Sage.

A very useful introductory to advanced text for evaluation researchers.

Phillips, E. & Pugh, D. (1995) *How to get a PhD: a handbook for students and their supervisors*, 2nd edn. Bristol: Open University Press.
An interesting British account of higher degree work.

Polgar, S. & Thomas, S. (1995) *Introduction to research in the health sciences*, 3rd edn. Melbourne: Churchill Livingstone.
What more can I say?

Rossi, P. & Freeman, H. (1993) *Evaluation: a systematic approach 5*, 5th edn. Thousand Oaks, CA: Sage.
A standard evaluation text.

Rudestam, K. & Newton, R. (1992) *Surviving your dissertation: a comprehensive guide to content and process*. Thousand Oaks, CA: Sage.
A useful American account of higher degree work.

St Leger, A.S., Schnieden, H. & Walsworth-Bell, J.P. (1992) *Evaluating health services' effectiveness*. Buckingham: Open University Press.
A useful book for health service evaluations.

Stewart, M., Tudiver, F., Bass, M., Dunn, E. & Norton, P. (1992) *Tools for primary care research*, vol. 2. Thousand Oaks, CA: Sage.
A further discussion of the epistemology of health/medical research.

Strauss, A. & Corbin, J. (1990) *Basics of qualitative research: grounded theory procedures and techniques*. Thousand Oaks, CA: Sage.
A good introductory qualitative text. Obviously, Corbin can write.

Streiner, D. & Norman, G. (1996). *Health measurement scales: a practical guide to their development and use*, 2nd edn. New York: Oxford University Press.
A more medical version of how to develop scales.

Usherwood, T. (1996) *Introduction to project management in health research: a guide for new researchers*. Buckingham: Open University Press.
A good little book on how to keep the threads ravelled.

Appendix: Thesis preparation checklist

Item	Notes	Outcome
Is the title informative and concise?	The reader should be able to discern the topic from the title. Avoid silly and colloquial titles.	
Does the abstract contain: • A clear statement of the topic in the first paragraph? • A rationale for the work being performed? • A discussion of the outcomes of the literature review? • A clear statement of the thesis aims/hypotheses? • A clear statement of the study/data collection(s) and how they have been conducted? • A clear statement of the study sample/participants? • A clear statement of the study outcomes? • A clear statement of what the contribution to knowledge has been?		
Does the introduction include: • A clear outline of the structure of the introduction? • A literature review in which all pertinent literature has been covered? • An appropriately critical stance in the review of the literature? • A clear discussion of the outcomes of the literature review including identification of knowledge gaps?		

Item	Notes	Outcome
• A rationale for the study drawing upon the literature review outcomes? • A clear statement of the study aims and hypotheses?		
Does the method section include: • A full description of how the study participants were chosen? • Details of how many study participants were approached and how many participated? • A full description of all tools and protocols used in the study including interview schedules, tools and apparatus? • A balanced methodological defence of the tools and methods chosen?		
Does the results chapter(s) contain: • A clear outline of the structure of the results chapter(s)? • Uniquely numbered tables and figures? • Table and figure titles that could be taken out of the document, shown to an intelligent layperson and their content understood? • Consistently formatted tables and figures prepared according to the relevant style standards?		
Does the discussion chapter include: • A clear outline of the structure of the discussion chapter? • A point by point analysis of how your results answer the research questions you presented in the thesis introduction?		

Item	Notes	Outcome
• A discussion of how your results compare to the rest of the literature reviewed in the literature review?		
Does the conclusion chapter include: • A clear outline of the structure of the conclusion chapter? • A short review of the studies you conducted in the thesis? • A clear description of the outcomes of the study you have performed? • A discussion of the strengths and weaknesses of the study you have performed? • A discussion of the future work that is suggested by your study outcomes?		
References • Are all the references cited in the text, included in the reference list? • Are all the references in the reference list included in the text? • Do all references adhere to the appropriate style conventions?		
Structure • Is there an accurate table of contents? • Is there an accurate list of figures and tables? • Are all appendices listed in the text included? • Have you included your ethics clearance details in the locally prescribed manner?		
Have you adhered to all local requirements for submission, e.g. • binding method • number of copies • 100 word summary?		

Item	Notes	Outcome
Have you provided your supervisors with copies of the thesis exactly as you submitted it?		

Index